15th J   1981

To Tom,

With best wishes &
happy memories,

Bob.

607312

A SHORT TEXTBOOK OF CLINICAL ONCOLOGY

University Medical Texts

General Editor
Selwyn Taylor D.M., M.CH. [OXON], F.R.C.S.

A Short Textbook of Medicine Sixth edition
J. C. Houston M.D., F.R.C.P.
C. L. Joiner M.D., F.R.C.P.
J. R. Trounce M.D., F.R.C.P.

A Short Textbook of Surgery Fourth edition
Selwyn Taylor D.M., M.CH., F.R.C.S.
L. T. Cotton M.CH., F.R.C.S.

A Short Textbook: Ear, Nose and Throat Second edition
R. Pracy M.B., F.R.C.S.
J. Siegler M.B., B.S., F.R.C.S., D.L.O.
P. M. Stell M.B., F.R.C.S.

A Short Textbook of Chemical Pathology Third edition
D. N. Baron M.D., D.SC., F.R.C.P., F.R.C.PATH.

A Short Textbook of Orthopaedics and Traumatology Second edition
J. N. Aston M.B., F.R.C.S.

A Short Textbook of Psychiatry Second edition
W. L. Linford Rees B.SC., M.D., F.R.C.P., D.C.M.

A Short Textbook of Venereology Second edition
R. D. Catterall F.R.C.P. [EDIN.]

A Short Textbook of Gynaecology and Obstetrics
G. D. Pinker M.D., F.R.C.S., F.R.C.O.G.
D. W. T. Roberts M.CHIR., F.R.C.S., F.R.C.O.G.

A Short Textbook of Paediatrics
P. Catzel M.D., B.CH., F.R.C.P., D.C.H.

A Short Textbook of Medical Statistics
Sir Austin Bradford Hill C.B.E., D.SC., PH.D., HON. D.SC. [OXON],
HON. M.D. [EDIN.], F.F.C.M. [HON.], F.R.C.P. [HON.], F.R.S.

A Short Textbook of Preventive Medicine for the Tropics
A. O. Lucas M.D., D.P.H., D.T.M. & H., F.R.C.P., S.M.HYG., F.M.C.P.H.
H. M. Gilles M.D., F.R.C.P., F.F.C.M., F.M.C.P.H., D.T.M. & H.

A Short Textbook of Medical Microbiology Fourth edition
D. C. Turk D.M., M.R.C.P., F.R.C.PATH.
I. A. Porter M.D., F.R.C.PATH.

A SHORT TEXTBOOK
OF
CLINICAL
ONCOLOGY

R. D. RUBENS
M.D., B.Sc., F.R.C.P.

*Consultant, Imperial Cancer Research Fund and
Honorary Consultant Physician
Guy's Hospital, London*

and

R. K. KNIGHT
M.B., F.R.C.P.

*Consultant Physician
Guy's Hospital, London*

SHODDER AND STOUGHTON
LONDON   SYDNEY   AUCKLAND   TORONTO

British Library Cataloguing in Publication Data

Rubens, R D
  A short textbook of clinical oncology. –
  (University medical texts).
  1. Cancer
  I. Title   II. Knight, R K   III. Series
  616.9'94   RC261

  ISBN 0–340–21908–4
  ISBN 0–340–21909–2 Pbk

Filmset by Northumberland Press Ltd, Gateshead, Tyne and Wear
Printed in Great Britain for
Hodder and Stoughton Educational,
Mill Road, Dunton Green, Sevenoaks, Kent
a division of Hodder and Stoughton Ltd,
by Biddles Ltd, Guildford, Surrey

EDITOR'S FOREWORD

When a branch of medicine develops so effectively and excitingly as to earn itself a new name, as has Clinical Oncology, it is clear it has come to stay. I think Edward Lear would have described oncology as a compendious word, derived as it is from the Greek *ogkos* meaning a mass or tumour and *logos*, science. Clinical Oncology is the application of this new knowledge to the treatment of patients with malignant disease and the advances made in this field in recent years appear astonishing to the older clinician. Such conditions as Hodgkin's disease and choriocarcinoma, which were invariably fatal a few years ago, are now usually curable or well controlled by present treatment and the growth of many other tumours has been checked

Although individual advances in treating particular tumours have occasionally been outstanding, it is the combined approach of surgery, radiotherapy, chemotherapy and hormone manipulation which has been the hallmark of success in clinical oncology. Cancer first shows itself in such a multitude of ways that a broad knowledge of medicine, surgery and pathology is a prerequisite for the doctor who would enter this field.

This short textbook is broad in both scope and outlook and I welcome it as an excellent guide to complement the other volumes in the series of University Medical Texts. The medical student, will I know, welcome its clarity and many practising doctors will find in its pages a succinct account of this exciting and rapidly expanding field. I hope to see a new edition within a few years and at regular intervals thereafter.

Royal Postgraduate Medical School
Hammersmith Hospital

Selwyn Taylor

PREFACE

Clinical oncology is an expanding speciality. In recent years considerable advances have been made both in the understanding of disorders of cell growth and in the management of malignant diseases. Comprehensive texts and authoritative monographs on cancer medicine exist but clinical oncology is not given sufficient coverage in most general medical textbooks. Our purpose is to try to provide the essential principles of this subject.

To understand the modern approach to cancer treatment it is essential to have some knowledge of the regulation of cell growth and its disorders and we begin with a brief account of these processes. Later, discussion on treatment emphasises the combined approach of surgery, radiotherapy and chemotherapy but we have avoided giving too much technical detail. We have suggested some further reading, but have made no attempt to orientate the reader into the vast literature in oncology as we believe that students requiring more information are best guided in direct discussion with specialists.

Since cancer can arise at any site, its manifestations are protean and patient management requires a broad knowledge of general medicine; we have paid special attention to this. It is hoped that this book will be useful to both undergraduates, and more experienced doctors interested in the subject, and also to nurses concerned with the care of patients with cancer.

We thank Professor J. R. Trounce for encouraging us to write this book and for his helpful comments and criticisms during the preparation of the manuscript. Our thanks are also given to Mr T. M. Coltart, Mr J. L. Hayward, Dr R. A. C. Hughes, Mr M. Joyce, Mr O. H. Shaheen, Dr G. E. Sladen, Dr M. N. H. Tattersall, Dr C. Terrell, Dr R. S. Wells and Mr A. K. Yates for advising us on the chapters dealing with subjects in which they have particular expertise. Finally, we wish to express our gratitude to Miss A. E. McArthur for the long hours of patient secretarial assistance she has given us and to Mrs B. Taylor and Mrs M. Thomas for additional help.

<table>
<tr><td>Guy's Hospital,
London
1980</td><td>R. D. Rubens
R. K. Knight</td></tr>
</table>

CONTENTS

PART 1
GENERAL PRINCIPLES

CHAPTER ONE

BIOLOGY OF CANCER

INTRODUCTION

The diseases called 'cancers' or 'malignant tumours' are the clinical results of disorders in the regulation of cell proliferation. Knowledge about how these disorders develop and their causation is fragmentary, but considerable advances in our understanding of the problem have been made in recent years.

Normal cell proliferation (often referred to incorrectly as 'cell growth') is dependent upon the accurate replication of deoxyribose nucleic acid (DNA) and subsequent mitosis. Abnormalities of DNA may arise as a result of either random replication errors (mutations) or damage by external agencies (e.g. X-rays, chemicals, viruses). If these abnormalities are not corrected by DNA repair enzymes, then the cells concerned either die or give rise to abnormal daughter cells. These abnormal cells may not respond normally to cell regulation mechanisms and consequently excessive proliferation may occur and a tumour result.

Tumours which comprise cells retaining the morphological characteristics of the normal cell (differentiated) and which remain localised in the body, often encapsulated, are called benign. **Oncology**, however, is the study of malignant tumours and these arise from cells which have varying degrees of differentiation and have the abilities to infiltrate surrounding normal tissue (invasion) and to separate from the original tumour mass (primary tumour) to form secondary tumours (metastases) elsewhere in the body, a process known as metastasis.

PATHOLOGY

The morbid anatomical features and the histopathological characteristics of tumours are well described in various textbooks of pathology and this subject will not be considered in detail here. A few general remarks, however, follow.

Certain generic names are used to describe tumours arising from different sites. The common cancers, for example those arising in the gastro-intestinal tract, lung and breast, arise from epithelial tissues and are known as carcinomas. This term is often qualified further according to the type of epithelium from which the tumour arises. Thus squamous epithelium gives rise to squamous-cell carcinomas, while glandular epithelium gives rise to adenocarcinomas. Tumours arising in mesenchymal tissues are called sarcomas and are similarly qualified depending on their site of origin (e.g. osteosarcoma, fibrosarcoma, liposarcoma). Certain tumours are given more specific names, for example, tumours arising in lymphatic tissue are called lymphomas. Other aspects of oncological nomenclature will be introduced in Part 2.

Histological features of tumours vary considerably in comparison to the normal tissues in which they develop. Should the tumour resemble closely the parent tissue it is said to be well differentiated, but if, on the other hand, there is little similarity, then it is referred to as poorly differentiated or anaplastic.

The mechanisms of the spread of tumours are poorly understood, but it is likely that invasion is a prerequisite for metastasis. However, some malignant tumours invade only the surrounding normal tissues and do not metastasise (e.g. basal-cell carcinomas of the skin). Tumours which do metastasise do so usually through lymphatics and blood vessels although other routes are sometimes involved (e.g. perineural, across serosal cavities). Some tumours have an initial tendency to metastasise through lymphatic channels (e.g. breast cancer, colon cancer) and when this occurs the first evidence of metastasis is in the regional lymph nodes. Tumours having this characteristic usually spread ultimately through the blood system to distant sites. Certain tumours, however, tend not to metastasise to regional lymph nodes and do so primarily through the blood stream (e.g. renal carcinoma).

Because malignant cells may spread to any part of the body, cancers can be associated with all types of disturbance of body function, and so in oncology the clinician sees a broad spectrum of clinical problems. Furthermore, because of the lack of cell differentiation that exists in many malignant tumours the cancer cells, due to derepression of gene function, may have properties not possessed by the parent tissue. Thus several tumours are characterised by the production of excessive quantities of substances in the body above the normal physiological levels. This is manifested clinically by ectopic endocrine syndromes or other non-metastatic manifestations of malignant disease so-called because the clinical features in these cases are not directly attributable to the physical presence of metastases.

CELL TRANSFORMATION

Much knowledge has been gained by observing the behaviour of cancer cells in culture. Cells can be maintained in a viable state, and often proliferate, in an artificial environment outside the body (*in vitro*). For their successful culture the cells must be in contact with a suitable medium which contains all the necessary nutrients, and exposed to appropriate concentrations of oxygen and carbon dioxide at the correct temperature.

Cells may be cultured either suspended in the medium or attached to the surface of the containing vessel.

Commonly, cells are cultured in flat Petri dishes. In such dishes cells derived from normal tissues grow attached to the floor of the dish in a single layer (monolayer), and cell proliferation and, therefore, expansion of the monolayer continues until the surface is covered, at which point proliferation stops (density-dependent inhibition of growth). Cancer cells, however, do not have such an orderly pattern of behaviour in culture and tend to proliferate to form a disorganised multilayer mass.

The term 'cell transformation' used in the experimental study of cancer refers to the transformation of cells having normal characteristics to ones with the abnormal, or malignant, characteristics described above. This term should not be confused with, and should be distinguished from, the term 'lymphocyte transformation' used in immunology which refers to the initiation of DNA synthesis by, and the subsequent division of, sensitised lymphocytes after exposure to the appropriate antigen.

Although cells of human origin can be cultured in the laboratory, the most commonly studied cells for *in vitro* experimentation are derived from mice and hamsters. Such cells can be transformed *in vitro* by small DNA viruses (polyoma and Simian virus 40). Elegant experiments have shown that this transformation is a consequence of the DNA of these viruses covalently binding to the DNA of the host's cells. When this happens, the virally derived DNA contributes to the genetic constitution of the cells and it is this newly acquired genetic information that confers on the cell its malignant properties. When such transformed cells are implanted into animals, tumours develop at the implantation site and may metastasise.

It has been known for many years that viruses containing ribo-nucleic acid (RNA) can also cause cell transformation and cancers to develop in animals, but until recently it was not understood how viral RNA could be incorporated into the genetic material of mammalian cells. The mystery was solved as a result of the discovery of RNA-directed DNA-polymerase (reverse transcriptase). This enzyme enables DNA to be transcribed from an RNA template, which is the converse of the transcription occurring normally in mammalian cells.

Although virally induced cell transformation is currently the best understood mechanism by which cells may become cancers, other cell-transforming agents are known. Certain chemicals (carcinogens) can cause normal cells to become transformed to the malignant type. For example, dimethylbenzanthracene causes mammary cancers in mice and liver cancers in rats. How these chemicals cause transformation is not known, but presumably they act either directly or indirectly on cellular DNA and effect a change in the genetic code after which malignant properties are conferred on the cell.

There is now much knowledge concerning the causation and mechanisms of cell transformation in experimental cancers, but much less is known about these fundamental processes in the development of human cancers. There is, however, some evidence that viruses, chemicals and other environmental factors may be involved in the aetiology of some human tumours (Chapter 2).

KINETICS OF CELL PROLIFERATION

Proliferating cells (both in normal tissue and in tumours) are conventionally referred to as passing through the cell cycle. The cell cycle comprises various phases (Fig. 1.1). The phase of mitosis during which a cell divides into two daughter cells is referred to as M phase. Following M phase there is a period during which cell metabolism continues, but in which there is no apparent activity directed towards further cell replication. This is known as the first post-mitotic gap or G_1 phase. At the end

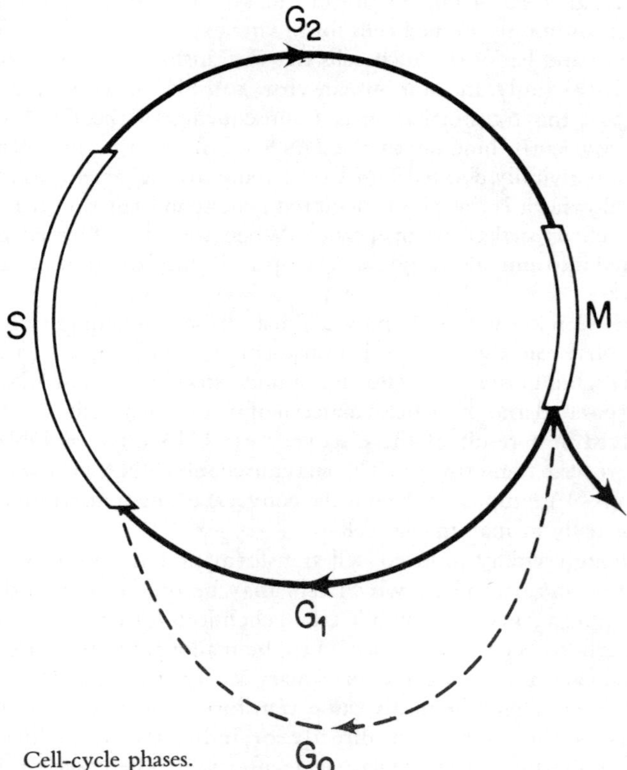

Fig. 1.1 Cell-cycle phases.

of G_1, DNA replication occurs, this is the DNA synthetic phase (S phase). The occurrence of the S phase commits the cell to subsequent mitosis but is followed by a second short post-mitotic gap (G_2 phase) before the next M phase. In certain cell populations, after mitosis has occurred, there is either no further cellular division (for example, in highly differentiated cell populations) or the G_1 phase is greatly prolonged because mitosis may not occur except under special circumstances (for example in healing tissues). Under these circumstances, the cell cycle ceases (G_0 phase).

Tumour growth is largely dependent upon two factors. The first is the proportion of cells undergoing cell-cycle activity, referred to as the growth fraction, and the second is the duration of the cell cycle. In experimental tumours much information concerning the kinetics of cell proliferation has been gained using thymidine labelled with radioactive hydrogen (tritiated thymidine). Only cells actively undergoing DNA synthesis incorporate this substance and can be studied by special photographic techniques (autoradiography). Our knowledge of the kinetics of human tumour growth is poor compared with that about experimental tumours. However, it is known that cell cycle times in the human and in experimental animals are similar but the growth fractions of human tumours are considerably less than those in experimental tumours. It is also known that the growth fraction of tumours is much higher in the early part of tumour growth when cell numbers are relatively low. As tumours enlarge in size, the growth fraction decreases. Thus a position in tumour growth is reached where there is exponential cell increase, but where the proportion of cells participating in this proliferation is continually diminishing. This may be described mathematically as a Gompertzian function which states that proliferation is at every instance exponential but with a growth constant that is simultaneously decreasing exponentially.

Tumour growth can also be expressed as volume doubling time and another factor which determines this is the cell death within the tumour. Thus a tumour may have a high growth fraction with a rapid proliferation but this may be counterbalanced by cell loss, and so the resulting tumour growth may be either slow or static. Conversely, if the growth fraction is small and the rate of cell loss is also low, the resultant tumour growth may be relatively rapid.

In summary, tumour growth depends upon:

(1) growth fraction.
(2) cell cycle time.
(3) cell loss.

The relevance of these kinetic considerations to therapy is discussed further in Chapter 5.

TUMOUR IMMUNOLOGY

Many different types of tumour cells have been shown to possess protein components which are not possessed by normal host cells. These abnormal constituents may be recognised by the host animal as foreign and, are, therefore, capable of initiating an immune reaction. These are known as tumour-associated antigens.

Tumours induced by viruses possess such antigens. Here the tumour-associated antigens are coded by viral nucleic acid, and, because they lead to rejection of these tumours when transplanted, are referred to as tumour-specific transplantation antigens (TSTA). When the same virus is able to transform different cell types it leads to the production of the same TSTA which are common to the transforming virus and not the type of cell transformed. In contrast, a tumour induced by a chemical carcinogen in an experimental animal possesses antigens unique to itself, while another tumour induced by the same chemical in an immunologically identical animal will have different antigens.

Cancer cells sometimes exhibit antigens present in embryonic tissues but which are not normally seen in the adult. These are embryonic or oncofoetal antigens, which are detectable in some cancers whether caused by viruses, chemicals or other unknown factors.

The two principal types of immune reaction, antibody formation and lymphocyte sensitisation (cell-mediated immunity), occur in response to tumour-associated antigens. Cell-mediated immunity is concerned with the rejection of tumours and this, therefore, has a protective function for the host. This type of reaction is analogous to the rejection of tissue transplants. Sometimes antibody production can be detrimental to the host and result in an enhancement of tumour growth. When this occurs it is probable that the binding of the antibody to the antigen prevents sensitised lymphocytes from binding to the same antigen, and, therefore prevents rejection. This phenomenon is known as blocking. However, in clinical cancer it appears that circulating antibodies are usually associated with a better prognosis, when they possibly bind tumour antigens shed from tumour tissue and prevent these antigens binding to cytotoxic immune lymphocytes leaving them free to reject tumour cells.

The precise role of immunity in the natural history of human cancer is still poorly understood, but there is evidence that it might be of considerable importance. As already mentioned, the demonstration of antibodies in human cancer is often associated with a better response to therapy and prognosis. Furthermore, the demonstration of immune reactivity in cancer patients against various test antigens is often associated with an improved prognosis. Lymphocytic infiltration in tumours is also a favourable factor.

Recent interest in tumour immunology has stimulated many in-

vestigations to study how antigenic peculiarities of malignant cells could
be exploited therapeutically (immunotherapy) and this will be discussed
in Chapter 4.

CHAPTER TWO

EPIDEMIOLOGY AND CAUSES OF HUMAN CANCER

EPIDEMIOLOGY

Epidemiology is the study of the distribution of diseases in human populations. This approach, which includes such factors as geographical distribution, variation in frequency at different times and the relationship of diseases to occupations, has, in the case of malignant diseases, shed more light on the causes of certain cancers than any other form of research. Furthermore, it leads to possible ways for the prevention of cancer and the organisation of health services to provide treatment.

Mortality statistics

Data on causes of death are derived from death certificates issued by doctors (e.g. Table 2.1). In most developed countries, malignant neoplasms are the second most common cause of death (Table 2.2), accounting for about 20 per cent of all deaths in the United Kingdom. The apparent increase in the number of deaths from cancer is, in part, due to such factors as an increase in the proportion of elderly people, eradication of other diseases and improved diagnostic facilities, but there has been a real increase in the incidence of some tumours (notably carcinoma of the bronchus).

Official statistics in the elderly, where investigation before death may have been curtailed, probably underestimate the incidence of cancer. Mortality rates are similar to incidence only in tumours which are not cured by treatment and cause death. The incidence of tumours which respond well to treatment (e.g. seminoma) or which seldom cause death (e.g. skin cancers) cannot be deduced from the mortality figures for these tumours. For this information and that concerning the prevalence of tumours in which treatment is improving, other data are required.

Morbidity statistics

Morbidity statistics are more difficult to obtain than those on mortality. The most important sources of information about malignant diseases are the cancer registries. In some countries, notably Denmark and Finland, and the state of Connecticut, U.S.A., the entire population has been covered by case registration of a high standard for several years, but in others there is selective registration only. In Britain, a national programme has existed since 1962. Such registries require notification of

TABLE 2.1 Deaths due to Malignant Neoplasms in England and Wales in 1975

Site or type	Deaths (all ages)			
	Number		Rate per million	
	Male	Female	Male	Female
Buccal cavity and Pharynx	972	628	41	25
Oesophagus	1 886	1 484	79	59
Stomach	6 983	5 000	291	198
Intestine (excluding rectum)	4 355	6 379	182	253
Rectum and rectosigmoid junction	3 247	2 856	135	113
Larynx	587	139	24	6
Trachea, bronchus and lung	26 104	6 782	1 089	269
Bone	244	197	10	8
Skin	517	612	22	24
Breast	82	11 637	3	461
Cervix uteri	0	2 143	0	85
Corpus uteri	0	1 452	0	58
Prostate	4 421	0	184	0
Other and unspecified	12 378	13 919	516	551
Leukaemia	1 753	1 441	73	57
Other lymphatic and haematopoietic	2 262	1 992	94	79

(*Source* Mortality Surveillance Office of Population Censuses and Surveys, Medical Statistics Division.)

TABLE 2.2 Percentage of all deaths due to common certified causes (England and Wales)

Coronary heart disease	25.9
Neoplasms	20.6
Cerebrovascular disease	13.7
Pneumonia	8.0
Chronic bronchitis	4.1
Accidents	3.8

(*Source* D. J. P. Barker and G. Rose, *Epidemiology in Medical Practice*, Churchill Livingstone, 1976.)

cancer patients and a record of the site and histological types of their tumours.

Information obtained in this way permits studies of cancer incidence and survival, and exposes some environmental hazards.

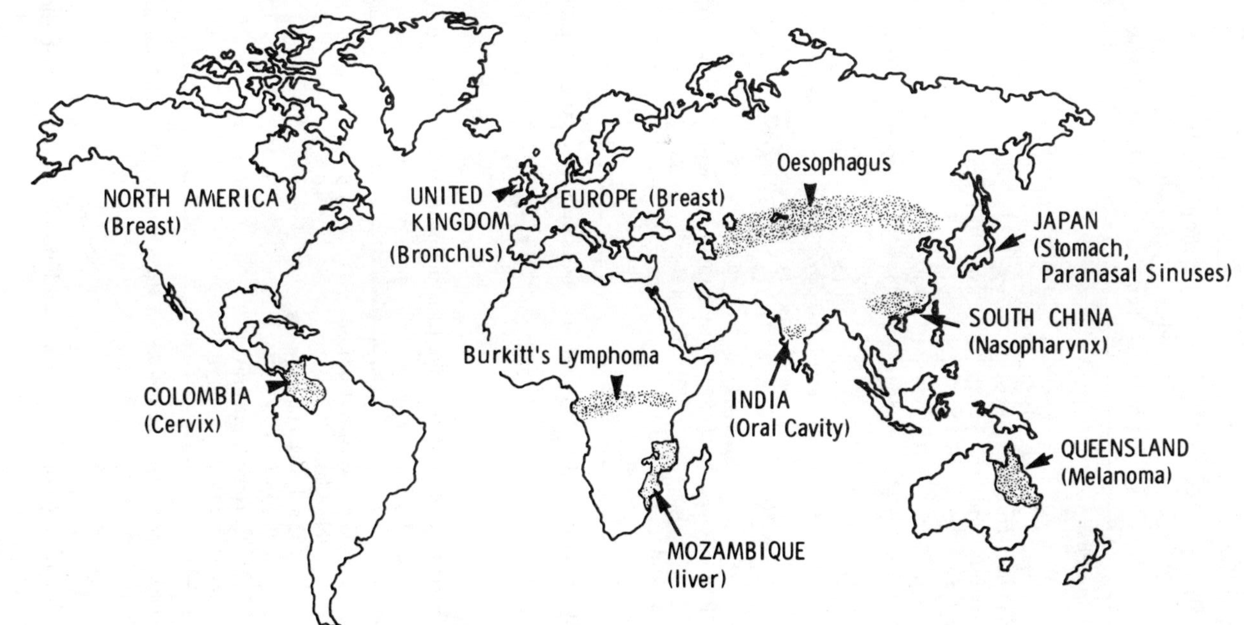

FIG. 2.1   World map showing areas where a very high incidence of certain tumours is found.

Geographical pathology

The relatively recent concept of geographical pathology is a form of epidemiology which recognises that while some tumours are distributed fairly uniformly throughout the world, others have a strikingly high incidence in certain areas (Fig. 2.1). Collecting data is difficult in some countries with incomplete records, but the technique may help to identify causes of certain neoplasms.

Some of the more remarkable instances of particular cancers occurring often in certain areas include oesophageal cancer near the Caspian Sea, Burkitt's lymphoma in Africa and New Guinea within a narrow range of temperature and rainfall, and primary liver tumours in South East Africa. These strongly suggest an environmental risk, although in some other instances genetic factors cannot be ruled out entirely. It is now known that migrant groups tend to acquire the pattern of incidence of their adopted countries, as in the case of Japanese women, who have a low incidence of breast cancer in Japan, but acquire a greater incidence after settling in Hawaii and greater still in California.

CAUSES OF CANCER

A number of physical or chemical agents are known to produce cancer in man, but the cause of the majority of human tumours is not known. The very long interval between exposure, which may not be prolonged and may have ceased, and the appearance of the cancer, makes it difficult to recognise the association.

Physical agents

Ionising radiation is one of the physical agents which has been known for many years to produce tumours in man. In the early days of radiology, people (especially doctors) coming into contact with X-rays either for diagnosis or therapy were prone to develop various tumours, particularly of the skin exposed to the radiation. The use of therapeutic X-rays for the treatment of ankylosing spondylitis produces a five-fold increase in acute leukaemia among the patients so treated, and even small doses associated with diagnostic X-rays are potentially hazardous for the foetus *in utero*, having been shown to increase the risk of leukaemia developing later. One of the most spectacular demonstrations of the risk of ionising radiation occurred after the atomic bombs were dropped on Hiroshima and Nagasaki in World War II when large numbers of the population were exposed to radiation and were carefully followed up afterwards. A marked increase in the incidence of leukaemia was noted in the following years. Miners who are exposed to radon gas during the mining of uranium, haematite or fluorspar have an increased incidence of carcinoma of the bronchus. A form of bone cancer used to be produced in women who painted the luminous dials on to watches and in doing so licked the brushes thereby absorbing radium.

Prolonged exposure to intense heat may in certain circumstances induce cancer. Some of the inhabitants of Kashmir keep themselves warm by carrying around under their clothing earthenware pots containing hot coals, a practice known as 'Kangri' and in due course this produces skin cancers on the abdomen and thighs. In certain parts of the world it is customary to smoke cigarettes with the lighted end in the mouth, and this may produce carcinoma of the palate.

Chemicals in industry

A number of chemicals are known to cause cancer and where these have been identified in industry, their use has either been prohibited or controlled. The oldest example of this is the scrotal cancer which occurred in chimney sweeps due to contact with 3-4 benzpyrene. Aromatic amines, which have been used in the rubber and dyestuffs industries, cause carcinoma of the bladder many years after exposure and these substances have now been withdrawn. People who work with asbestos and particularly those involved with certain mining procedures are liable to an increased risk of carcinoma of the bronchus, and with a particular form of asbestos, Crocidolite, there is a risk of pleural or peritoneal mesothelioma. Other workers who handle asbestos fibre, in the lagging of boilers and pipes or those who cut, saw or drill asbestos material, may also be exposed to such a risk and indeed, asbestos is now so ubiquitous that many people handle it outside the industries where conditions are controlled, which poses a much wider hazard. In the chemical industry during the manufacture of chromates or in the refining of nickel ore there was a hazard of an increased incidence of carcinoma of the bronchus. Certain furniture makers who work with hard-wood are prone to develop carcinoma of the nasal sinuses, although the exact constituent of the wood dust which is responsible is not known.

Drugs

Although in recent years new drugs have only been allowed on the market after very careful scrutiny, there are some which are known to carry a risk of carcinogenesis. The use of oestrogens during pregnancy carries a risk of causing carcinoma of the vagina in female offspring and in adult women oestrogens may also be associated with increased risk of carcinoma of the corpus uteri. Immunosuppressive drugs used after transplantation surgery are known to be associated with an increased risk of lymphomas and other tumours.

Cultural hazards

People who live in areas of the world where there is plenty of sunlight and who habitually expose themselves to it have an increased risk of cancers of the skin. In some areas in the East, it is customary to chew betel nuts, and this is associated with the development of tumours in the mouth. Certain forms of alcohol are known to be associated with increased incidence of carcinoma of the oesophagus and the world-wide practice of smoking carries with it the well-known association with carcinoma of the bronchus and other tumours in the upper respiratory tract, oesophagus and bladder.

Viruses

Much speculation surrounds the role of viruses in human cancer, although this is probably small. The ability of viruses to produce tumours in laboratory animals is well established and has been known for more than 60 years. RNA viruses can induce lymphomas, leukaemia and sarcomas in several animals, including chickens, mice and cats. Some viruses with DNA genomes have been found to be carcinogenic, producing malignant transformation of normal cells in tissue culture and certain tumours when injected into laboratory animals. Marek's disease in chickens is caused by a herpes virus and an effective vaccine against it now exists—the first example of a common, naturally occurring tumour controllable by an anti-viral vaccine.

Notwithstanding these observations and the extensive research in this field, there is so far no proof that viruses cause cancer in man. Suggestive evidence, however, is particularly strong with regard to the association of the Epstein–Barr virus with Burkitt's lymphoma and perhaps also with a herpes simplex virus in carcinoma of the cervix. It is likely that further evidence will be forthcoming before very long, but viruses, if they do account for any human tumours, probably do so for a relatively small number.

Environmental hazards

In addition to those chemical hazards already mentioned there exist undoubtedly a number of environmental hazards, some of which are known, but the majority of which are only suspected. Epidemiological studies suggest strongly that environmental factors play a very important part in the development of human cancers and may well account for up to 90 per cent of all tumours. Research in this field is of the utmost importance since identification of these agents is the most likely way in which certain tumours may in the future be prevented.

CHAPTER THREE

ASSESSMENT OF THE CANCER PATIENT

The definitive diagnosis of cancer depends upon the histological examination of tumour tissue, but it is essential that patients are carefully assessed in order to determine, as precisely as possible, the extent of the tumour within the body. This assessment, at the time of diagnosis, provides a baseline on which to plan and, subsequently, monitor treatment. Furthermore, because most cancer treatments cannot at the present time be considered optimal, many patients are treated in therapeutic trials (Chapter 4) and an accurate baseline examination and subsequent assessments are essential in the evaluation of cancer therapies.

History

Of first importance is the recording of a detailed history. This should provide information on several different, but closely related, aspects about the patients. The evolution of symptoms due directly to the tumour should be studied as these give important information about the duration and extent of disease. Furthermore, certain symptoms may have important prognostic implications, for example the 'B' symptoms (weight loss, fever and night sweats) in Hodgkin's disease (Chapter 10). Past illnesses and medication should be noted as these may be related aetiologically to the cancer (e.g. radiation therapy for ankylosing spondylitis and subsequent leukaemia) or be of relevance in planning treatment. Occupational and environmental history should be noted with care, particularly regarding previous exposure to potential carcinogenic substances. Family history too is of particular relevance to several cancers.

An estimation of a patient's physical ability should be made and this can be expressed conveniently as a performance grading as follows:*

Grade 0   fully active, able to carry on all usual activities without restriction and without the aid of analgesia;

Grade 1   restricted in strenuous activity but ambulatory and able to carry out light work or pursue a sedentary occupation. This group also contains patients who are fully active, as in grade 0, but only with the aid of analgesics;

Grade 2   ambulatory, capable of all self-care but unable to work.

* Recommended by the International Union Against Cancer, *British Journal of Cancer*, (1977). **35**, 292.

Up and about more than 50 per cent of waking hours;

Grade 3   capable of only limited self-care. Confined to bed or chair more than 50 per cent of waking hours;

Grade 4   completely disabled, unable to carry out any self-care and confined totally to bed or chair.

Physical examination

A full physical examination must be carried out, careful attention being given not only to the primary tumour, its extent and dissemination, but also to other tissues or organs where toxic manifestations of subsequent treatment might be expected to develop. It is important to recognise the presence of other associated conditions which may require treatment or affect the feasibility of specific anticancer therapy. General features to be noted on physical examination include evidence of weight loss, skin colour abnormality (e.g. jaundice, anaemia), the presence of clubbing and the psychological state with special reference to anxiety, fear and depression. Other associated clinical features of the various cancers will be outlined in more detail in Part 2.

Superficial and palpable lesions should be measured directly along two axes (one being the longest axis and, the other, the longest perpendicular to it); callipers may improve the accuracy of these measurements. Visible lesions should be photographed. Lesions particularly suitable for serial assessment by physical examination are skin and subcutaneous nodules and superficial lymph-node involvement. Infiltration of tissues by tumour can be assessed by measurement, but this is sometimes difficult. It is feasible for diffuse involvement of breast tissue which can be measured after compressing the breast digitally between two marks centred on the nipple; comparison may be possible with similar measurements on a contralateral normal breast. Similarly, lymphoedema may be measured with reference to fixed points on a limb and compared with an unaffected contralateral limb.

Involvement of the liver in malignant disease often leads to hepatic enlargement and this may be measured by determining the vertical distance of the inferior edge of the liver from the costal margin. For subsequent measurements to be comparable, the exact point at, or lateral to, the midline at which the liver was palpated should be recorded, as should the phase of respiration (quiet breathing or deep inspiration). Ascites may be assessed by periodical measurement of abdominal girth and body weight, and abdominal masses may sometimes be sufficiently defined for measurements to be taken. The presence of serous effusions in the pleural and pericardial spaces (Chapter 20) may also be determined on examination, but their assessment is more appropriately done radiographically. Neurological examination gives information about malignant involvement of the nervous system and also the presence of non-metastatic neurological manifestations of cancer (Chapter 17).

Investigations

After the first clinical evaluation of a patient suspected of having malignant disease, further investigations will be necessary, generally including a biopsy procedure. The order in which investigations should be carried out depends upon the type of disease present and the information gained at the first clinical assessment. The appropriate selection of investigations will be elaborated upon further in the discussion of the individual tumours (Part 2); only a brief summary of the types of available investigations will be given here.

A full blood count including estimation of haemoglobin, white blood cells and platelets is usually required, and microscopic examination of the bone marrow, after either aspiration or biopsy, is often needed, particularly with haematological malignancies and lymphomas. A biochemical screen should include estimation of blood urea and/or creatinine, serum bilirubin, liver transaminases, alkaline phosphatase, calcium, uric acid and plasma proteins. This screen provides general information on renal and liver function as well as possible complications of malignant disease (hepatic metastases, hypercalcaemia, hyperuricaemia). Elevated alkaline phosphatase in a cancer patient may be due to an osteoblastic reaction to metastases in bone, involvement of the liver or inappropriate production of this enzyme by the tumour (particularly carcinoma of the bronchus). It is possible to differentiate between these causes by isoenzyme studies of alkaline phosphatase. Other biochemical tests sometimes of value include serum acid phosphatase (usually elevated in metastatic prostatic cancer) and serum amylase (elevated in 25 per cent of cases of carcinoma of the pancreas). There are various other substances on which research is being done which may be of importance, in the future, in detecting and monitoring the response of cancer to treatment. These so-called 'biological markers' include the foetal proteins carcino-embryonic antigen and alpha foeto-protein. At the present time the most specific marker available is chorionic gonadotrophin for choriocarcinoma where it is invaluable in guiding the management of this condition.

Radiographic examinations are of particular value in assessing the cancer patient. A plain radiograph of the chest (postero-anterior and lateral views) is essential to assess the extent and position of a tumour in the thorax and other plain radiographs of value are of the bones and breasts (mammography). The use of contrast media is important in the investigation of many tumours, particularly the alimentary tract, urinary tract and lymph nodes (lymphography); contrast arteriography of several tumours may give valuable information. Tomograms are useful in certain situations, particularly in assessing the extent of pulmonary, mediastinal and laryngeal tumours.

The uptake of substances labelled with radioactive isotopes can be used to investigate many tumours, being detected by either a rectilinear scanner or gamma camera. Increased uptake of an isotope may be due to the avidity of the tumour for a particular substance (e.g. iodine in thyroid cancer, gallium in Hodgkin's disease), or simply a reflection of the increased vascularity of the tumour. Conversely, decreased uptake of an isotope may indicate the presence of relatively avascular tumour tissue as with most hepatic metastases.

Certain non-invasive radiological investigations have achieved a high degree of accuracy, particularly the chest radiograph, tomography, barium studies, urography and cholecystography. However, there are some anatomical regions in which radiography does not provide adequate definition when non-invasive procedures only are used (e.g. mediastinum, liver, pancreas, central nervous system and lymphatic system). There has therefore been considerable interest in the development of computerised tomography (CT scanning), in which sections of the body are scanned by an X-ray beam in multiple planes sequentially, and the X-ray absorption at numerous positions is detected and processed by a computer. The computed body anatomy can then be displayed on a cathode-ray tube and photographed as a permanent record. The intravenous injection of certain contrast media can further increase the definition of lesions seen by this technique. CT scanning is now well-established in the investigation of intracranial lesions (Chapter 17) and the use of the invasive techniques of cerebral arteriography and air encephalography are consequently used much less. It is likely that in future years this technique will become further established and have extensive application in the investigation and management of cancer patients.

Ultrasonic scanning of the abdomen is helpful in the detection and, sometimes, measurement of visceral swellings such as hepatic and pancreatic tumours. This technique involves the use of very high-frequency sound waves the reflection of which from surfaces within the body is recorded by detectors and processed to give a visual display. With increasing refinement this method is likely to pay a bigger role in the assessment of tumours within the abdomen.

Many parts of the body can be visualised directly by endoscopic techniques. Older rigid instruments are being replaced by flexible fibre-optic instruments and the whole alimentary system, with the exception of the jejunum and ileum, can now be visualised. In addition the ampulla of Vater can be cannulated at duodenoscopy, and contrast media injected retrogradely into the pancreatic and bile ducts for radiographic examination. Other useful endoscopic investigations include cystoscopy, laparoscopy and laryngoscopy.

Adequate biopsy of a tumour to obtain tissue for the definitive histological diagnosis is essential in the management of all cancers. For superficial lesions (e.g. skin nodule, lymph node), this is readily done by incision or excision biopsy, but sometimes a needle biopsy is preferred and this technique can also be used to acquire tissue from several internal lesions (lung, pleura, liver, bone marrow). Biopsy is readily performed during endoscopy with many tumours, but for some cancers this must be done at a major operation such as thoracotomy or laparotomy. Examination under anaesthetic is also useful in assessing the extent of certain tumours, particularly in the head and neck region and the pelvis. Dilatation of the cervix and curretage is an important procedure in the diagnosis of uterine cancer.

Cytological examination may give initial information indicating the malignant nature of a certain disease, this type of investigation being readily done on the uterine cervix, sputum, effusions, urine and cerebro-spinal fluid.

Staging

After a full clinical assessment of the cancer patient has been carried out, and the diagnosis confirmed, it is then usual practice to stage a tumour before planning treatment. Various staging systems are available for different tumours and these will be discussed in more detail in Part 2. The object of staging is to guide the selection of appropriate treatment and give an indication of prognosis. A staging system should take into account the extent of the primary tumour, involvement of regional lymph nodes and distant metastases. In the TNM system, developed by the International Union against Cancer, the primary tumour is designated 'T' to which a numbered suffix is added to indicate the extent of the primary tumour. Regional lymph nodes ('N') are similarly suffixed, while 'M_0' signifies the absence of distant metastases and 'M_1' means their presence. As an example, a breast cancer may be described as $T_{3b} \, N_2 \, M_0$. This indicates that the tumour is greater than 5 cm in diameter and fixed deeply, the axillary nodes are palpable and fixed to one another or to surrounding structures, and there is no evidence of distant metastases. The TNM system thus provides a shorthand notation to describe a malignant tumour.

Assessment of response to therapy

An accurate evaluation of a patient must be made whenever a new treatment is started in order to provide a baseline on which the response to this treatment can be assessed. The generally accepted categories of response are as follows:

1 **Objective Regression.**
  (a) *complete response:* this means the disappearances of all known disease determined by two observations not less than four weeks apart.
  (b) *partial response:* For this response to have been achieved there must have been a 50 per cent or more decrease in the size of measurable lesions and also an objective improvement in evaluable but non-measurable lesions (e.g. lesions being assessed by photography or

radiography), with no new lesions developing, determined by two observations not less than four weeks apart.

2 No Change.
Disease is considered to be unchanged if there is a less than 50 per cent decrease or a less than 25 per cent increase in the size of measurable lesions.

3 Progressive Disease.
(a) *mixed:* this applies when some lesions regress, but others progress in size or new lesions appear;
(b) *failure:* this means progression of some or all lesions and/or the appearance of new lesions without regression of any lesions.

When an objective regression has been achieved the duration of the overall response is dated from the start of therapy until either new lesions appear or any one existing lesion increases by 25 per cent or more above the smallest size recorded. The period of complete response is from the date the complete response was first recorded to the date of first observation of progressive disease. The length of survival on treatment should also be noted and dated from the time of commencement of treatment to death. In clinical trials it is recommended that the clinical records of all patients should be reviewed by independent external assessors in order to validate the findings of the investigators before they are published.

REFERENCES

M. H. Harmer (ed.), *TNM Classification of Malignant Tumours*, International Union against Cancer, 3rd edn, Geneva, 1978.

CHAPTER FOUR

PRINCIPLES OF CANCER TREATMENT

INTRODUCTION

The aim of treatment in patients with cancer is either cure, or, if this is not possible or fails, effective palliation. Sometimes long-term control of the disease by continuous treatment may be practicable.

In the curative approach, the treatment plan is to eradicate the cancer completely as soon as possible after the histological diagnosis has been made and the tumour accurately staged (Chapter 3). For effective and rational curative treatment, a knowledge of the precise histology of the tumour and its staging is of the utmost importance. The traditional approach to the primary treatment of localised tumours has been to attempt surgical resection, or, if this is not technically feasible, local radiotherapy; only when evidence of dissemination had occurred were systemic methods of treatment employed. However, it is becoming increasingly recognised that many cancers which present as localised disease eventually become widespread. For this reason the sequential use of different forms of treatment is gradually being replaced by the planned incorporation of systemic with local therapy at the time of diagnosis. The advances being made by the combined treatment approach will be discussed in the section on the individual tumours (Part 2).

The palliative approach to treatment is used either when it is known that the chance of cure is negligible, or if extensive curative treatment is inappropriate for other reasons, for example in an ill, elderly patient. In palliative treatment, prolongation of patient survival and tumour regression may or may not be achieved, but the principal aim is to achieve symptomatic relief (Chapter 23) and so improve the patient's quality of life. Certain cancers have extremely protracted courses and respond to treatment although the tumour cells are never eradicated entirely. These diseases are analogous to other chronic medical conditions (for example diabetes mellitus or hypertension), when many years of good quality life can be achieved by treatment, although the disease is not cured.

SURGERY

Surgery has had an established role in the treatment of cancer for centuries, and until this century there was indeed no other effective treatment. Furthermore, it is nearly always needed for diagnosis. Biopsy procedures for the histological classification of tumours are essential for rational treatment, and other operative procedures may be of importance in staging the disease (for example laparotomy in Hodgkin's disease; Chapter 10).

In planning surgery for the curative treatment of cancer, a knowledge of a tumour's individual behaviour with regard to local invasion and distant metastasis is vital. This knowledge helps ensure that the extent of surgery will be adequate so that sufficient tissue surrounding the tumour is removed, and, if appropriate, the draining lymphatic channels and regional lymph nodes removed in continuity with the tumour ('en bloc' dissection). Knowledge of the behaviour of the tumour will also temper attempts at extensive and ill-advised radical surgery if the likelihood of distant metastases is great, and the patient can be spared unpleasant and mutilating procedures when it is known that no benefit can be conferred, either from the point of view of quality of life or length of survival.

Surgery also has an important role to play in the treatment of advanced disease. The excision of a local recurrence near the primary operation site or in the regional lymph nodes, or occasionally the excision of a single metastasis from the brain or lung, may lead to a long period of disease-free survival or even cure. Palliation of other forms of advanced disease can be effectively achieved by surgery, for example the removal of a fungating breast mass or the resection or by-pass of a tumour causing intestinal obstruction. Orthopaedic surgical procedures may be of value in treating or preventing fractures at sites of metastases in bone. Surgical removal of endocrine organs can confer considerable benefit in patients with endocrine-dependent tumours (see below). Surgery may also have a diagnostic role in advanced cancer, for example to see whether a change in histology has occurred during the natural history of a cancer (e.g. with lymphomas), or in the excision of tissue for tests to give predictive information on whether a tumour is likely to benefit from other systemic therapy (e.g. oestrogen receptor analysis in advanced breast cancer; Chapter 8).

RADIOTHERAPY

Radiotherapy is the application of ionising radiations in the treatment of cancer. Such radiation causes tissue destruction and the therapeutic effectiveness of radiotherapy depends upon both the sensitivity of the cancer to irradiation and the susceptibility of normal surrounding tissues. The technical aspects of radiotherapy are complex, and a complete understanding of it requires a considerable knowledge of radiation physics; a detailed consideration of these aspects of radiotherapy is not appropriate here.

Radiotherapy is usually given in the form of X-irradiation. This can either be at low voltage from conventional X-ray equipment, or high voltage using a linear accelerator or a radioactive cobalt unit. Radioactive isotopes may also be administered in the treatment of certain tumours, for example iodine (^{131}I) for thyroid cancer and phosphorus (^{32}P) for polycythaemia rubra vera. Other forms of ionising radiation are now being studied in the treatment of cancer, for example neutrons, electrons and pi-mesons, but these are still experimental. The equipment needed for radiotherapy is heavy, immobile and expensive and is necessarily limited to certain specialised units. The logistics of administering radiotherapy are complex and treatment is usually given in repeated low doses until a planned total dose has been given (fractionation).

Radiotherapy has a curative role in a limited number of tumours (e.g. Stage I and II Hodgkin's disease, seminoma, rodent ulcer) and has an important role in the treatment of inoperable tumours when cures can be achieved occasionally. Radiotherapy is of considerable value in treating metastatic disease (e.g. in the skeleton and brain), and has an important role in combination with chemotherapy in treating systemic cancers (e.g. cranio-spinal irradiation in acute lymphoblastic leukaemia: Chapter 9).

Radiotherapy often produces side effects. If large volumes of bone marrow are irradiated the production of blood cells may be impaired. This can cause infections from leukopenia or lead to haemorrhage from thrombocytopenia; effects which may compromise subsequent chemotherapy. It is possible that suppression of lymphocyte function may produce immune deficiencies which will adversely affect host resistance to the tumour (Chapter 1). Administration of radiotherapy may be accompanied by malaise, nausea and vomiting, the incidence of which depends largely on the sites irradiated and the doses given. Normal tissues, other than bone marrow, can be damaged by irradiation. This is particularly so for skin at the portal of entry of the radiation. Skin reactions are more severe with low-voltage irradiation when the main ionising effect is at the skin surface, while this is less marked with megavoltage irradiation when the maximal ionisation is deep to the epidermis. Various techniques are used to distribute irradiation in normal tissues and direct them principally to the tumour so that there is relative sparing of normal tissues from these effects. Other tissues particularly liable to be damaged by irradiation are the lungs and kidneys and appropriate lead shielding of the organs must be given if these organs would otherwise be in the field of irradiation.

There is much interest in substances which increase the sensitivity of tumours to the effects of ionising radiation. Among these the promising ones include the use of hyperbaric oxygen and certain drugs, for example metronidazole.

SYSTEMIC THERAPY

Endocrine Therapy

The growth of some tumours is partly dependent upon hormones. This is particularly so with carcinomas of the breast, body of uterus and prostate. For these tumours circulating hormones have a permissive effect on their growth and antagonism or removal of these hormones may lead to a regression of tumour growth. This can be achieved either by removing the source of the stimulating hormone (e.g. oophorectomy in oestrogen-dependent breast cancers) or by administering other hormones having an effect opposite to that of the stimulating hormone (e.g. administration of androgens in oestrogen-dependent breast cancers). When endocrine therapy results in tumour regression, the effect is usually temporary because cells within the tumour which are relatively hormone independent eventually become the predominant proliferating cells, the tumour then becoming resistant to endocrine therapy. Endocrine therapy will be discussed further in the relevant chapters in Part 2.

Chemotherapy

Treatment of malignant tumours by drugs which inhibit cell proliferation (cytotoxic drugs) is having an expanding role in cancer medicine. Until recently such drugs were used only in the treatment of advanced disseminated malignancies, but they are now being used in the planned initial treatment of some cancers. The principles of chemotherapy and the pharmacology of the drugs are discussed in Chapter 5.

Immunotherapy

Immunotherapy in cancer medicine attempts to exploit antigenic peculiarities of malignant cells (Chapter 1). Immunotherapy can be divided into two types. First, the transfer of immunity from one individual to another either as antibodies (passive immunotherapy) or as immune lymphocytes (adoptive immunotherapy) or, secondly, by stimulating the immune mechanisms of the tumour-bearing host to reject the tumour (active immunotherapy). Attempts at passive and adoptive immunotherapy in treating human cancers have met with little success and have been associated with hypersensitivity reactions. These forms of immunotherapy have largely been abandoned.

Active immunotherapy has shown a little more promise and currently is being investigated in many research centres. Active immunotherapy can either be specific, when vaccines are prepared from the host's tumour cells, or non-specific, when immunity is stimulated by such agents as Bacille-Calmette-Guérin (BCG) or *Corynebacterium parvum*. A theoretical danger of active immunotherapy is that an excess of blocking antibody may be produced resulting in tumour enhancement (see Chapter 1). This, however, appears to be an infrequent occurrence with human cancers. It is improbable that immunotherapy alone will ever be capable of eradicating clinically established cancer because of the magnitude of antigen excess. Its role is more likely to be in eliminating residual tumour cells after the main bulk of tumour has been removed by other means. At the present time, immunotherapy must be regarded as a research procedure undergoing evaluation.

COMBINED TREATMENTS

Many cancers cannot be treated adequately simply by using only one of the treatment methods outlined above, and it is often expedient to combine therapies. This combined approach to the treatment of individual tumours will be considered when appropriate in Part 2.

CLINICAL TRIALS

The treatment of most cancers falls short of ideal. When new treatments are introduced, their true value should be established scientifically in controlled clinical trials, in which a new treatment is compared either with an existing treatment or with none in similar groups of patients.

In order to eliminate bias by observers and to prevent selection which would invalidate clinical trial observations, patients should be allocated at random to the treatment groups under study. Furthermore, placebos may be used when an inactive substance is given to one group under study in place of 'no treatment'. This inactive substance is apparently identical to the new treatment being tested (e.g. in appearance and flavour). When the patient is unaware of the preparation he is receiving the study is referred to as 'single-blind' and when, in addition, the clinical observers are unaware of the preparation it is a 'double-blind' study. Often however, it is not possible to do blind studies, as the agents under test have various side-effects, not possessed by placebos.

The results of new treatments are sometimes evaluated by comparing them with results achieved in the past by established therapies. Such studies are retrospective and the control groups are referred to as 'historical'. In these historically controlled studies, true comparability cannot be ensured for several reasons. First, patient selection can lead to considerable bias of results, secondly, assessment methods may change with time and, thirdly it is possible that the natural history of a disease may change with time, possibly influenced by environmental changes which may not be apparent. In order to obtain unequivocal information from clinical trials these studies should be prospective, when groups of patients are observed prospectively after being allocated randomly to the treatment groups under test as outlined above.

Clinical trials should be assessed from several points of view. Objective responses and their duration should be noted using well-defined criteria as described in Chapter 3. Although patient survival is an important index, the quality of life during this period and the toxicity of the treatment should also be carefully assessed. It is essential that the results of clinical trials are analysed statistically so that their significance can be determined. An excellent, lucid account of the design and analysis of clinical trials is given by Peto *et al.*, *British Journal of Cancer* (1976) **34** 585–612 and (1977) **35** 1–39.

GENERAL MEDICAL MANAGEMENT

The principles outlined in this chapter have been concerned with the specific treatment of malignant disease. However, many medical problems affect the cancer patient which are not necessarily attributable directly to the physical presence of the tumour mass. The management of these problems is discussed in Part 3.

CHAPTER FIVE

CANCER CHEMOTHERAPY

Although many malignant tumours present clinically as localised tumour masses, local therapy, either by surgery or radiotherapy, often fails to eradicate the disease because the process of metastasis has occurred before the primary tumour has become clinically apparent. This is illustrated graphically in Fig. 5.1. It is seen that if the metastatic process occurred before the primary tumour became evident, then the remission achieved by local treatment alone lasts only until metastases have grown to clinical proportions. Thus many malignant diseases are disseminated long before this is obvious clinically, and in these circumstances, if there is to be a chance of tumour eradication, then systemic therapy is required. More often, however, in practice, such treatment has been used for the temporary control of advanced disease.

Cytotoxic drugs are agents which inhibit the mechanisms of cell proliferation and are toxic, therefore, to both tumour cells and proliferating normal cells, particularly in the bone marrow, gastro-intestinal epithelium and hair follicles. However, there is some specificity against malignant tumours because a particularly high proportion of the component cells are undergoing division. Malignant tumours are, therefore, said to have a high *growth fraction*. Normal proliferating tissues, however, have a high percentage of non-dividing (resting) stem cells. The importance of this difference between normal and neoplastic cell populations will be discussed later in this chapter.

The first tumour ever to be cured by chemotherapy was choriocarcinoma. This is a rare disease, but information gained from the chemotherapy of this tumour, as well as of other rare malignancies (Burkitt's lymphoma, acute lymphoblastic leukaemia and Hodgkin's disease) have served as a basis from which the principles of modern chemotherapy are derived.

CYTOTOXIC DRUGS

Alkylating agents

Alkylating agents are highly reactive substances which are able to replace hydrogen atoms in other molecules by alkyl radicals. They are rapidly hydrolysed in aqueous solutions and their half-life in the body is short. The agents described here, except busulphan, are related to nitrogen mustard (Fig. 5.2). They possess two alkylating arms in the molecule

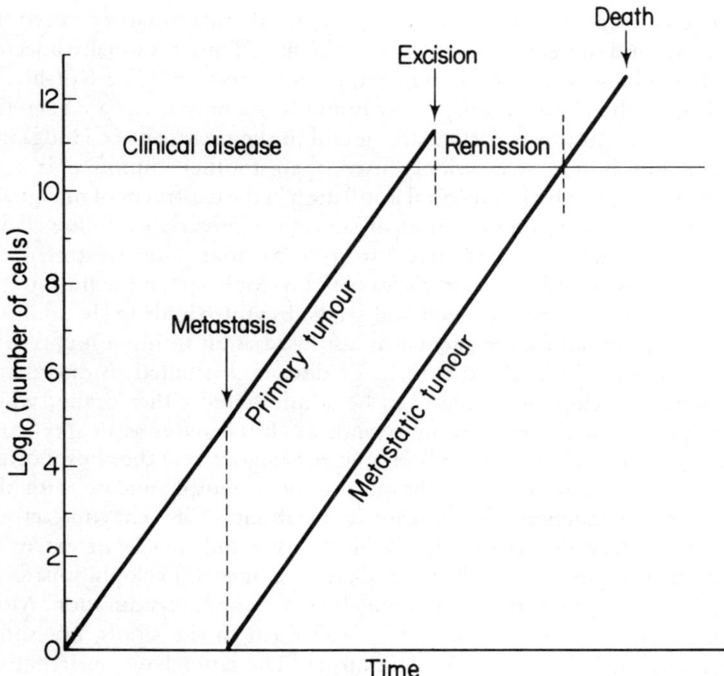

Fig. 5.1 Hypothetical model of exponential growth of a primary tumour arising from a single cancerous cell and the growth of a single cell which has metastasised during the pre-clinical growth of the tumour, illustrating the frequent incurability of cancer by local excision alone.

and are therefore termed *bifunctional alkylating agents*. Their mode of action as anticancer agents is attributed to an ability to react with the bases in deoxyribose nucleic acid (DNA), thereby cross-linking the two strands of the double helix. Resistance to these agents may develop as a consequence of enzymic excision of the alkylated groups (DNA repair), but other mechanisms of resistance may be involved, such as impairment of drug transport across cell membranes.

Nitrogen mustard (mustine). This is the most highly reactive of the alkylating agents. It is available in a crystalline form and is dissolved in water before injection. It must be given parenterally and prepared immediately before use as it is rapidly inactivated once in aqueous solution. The usual route of administration for systemic use is intravenous. It is essential for the drug to be administered directly into a vein as any subcutaneous extravasation causes a severe local inflammatory reaction, blistering, and subsequent ulceration of the skin. Thus it is usually injected into the tubing of a fast-running intravenous infusion. The half-life of the drug in the plasma is only a few minutes and only traces are excreted in the urine. Mustine is particularly useful in the treatment of Hodgkin's disease, but is not now widely used against other tumours. It can, however, be given by intrapleural instillation in the treatment of malignant pleural effusions. Administration of mustine is invariably followed by nausea and vomiting which may last up to 24 hours after treatment.

Cyclophosphamide (cytoxan, Endoxana). Cyclophosphamide (Fig. 5.3) is probably the most widely used and studied cytotoxic drug. In addition to its use as an anticancer agent it is also used as an immunosuppressive agent, particularly in the treatment of diseases attributed to disordered immunity. Cyclophosphamide can be administered either orally, when 70–80 per cent is absorbed, or intravenously. It is inactive as an alkylating agent until the cyclic group has been split enzymatically at the phosphorus–nitrogen linkage by either a phosphatase or a phosphamidase with the subsequent production of several active metabolites. This enzymic activation of the drug occurs principally in the liver and to a lesser extent in the plasma. Compared with other alkylating agents, cyclophosphamide has a long half-life in the plasma which is of some hours duration. Most of the drug is excreted in a metabolised form in the stools, but some metabolites are also excreted in the urine. The latter have an irritating effect on the transitional epithelium of the bladder, and may cause a chemical (and sometimes haemorrhagic) cystitis. This may be avoided by a high fluid intake. Cyclophosphamide administration may be associated with nausea, vomiting and the development of alopecia. These effects are more troublesome when the drug is given in high dosages intravenously, rather than by continuous low-dose oral administration. The drug is extensively used in a wide variety of malignant diseases.

Chlorambucil (Leukeran). This drug (Fig. 5.4) is the phenylbutyric derivative of nitrogen mustard. The aromatic radical decreases the reactivity of this alkylating agent. Chlorambucil is generally administered orally, but its sodium salt is soluble in water so that it may be used parenterally. Its metabolism and excretion are poorly understood. The principal uses of chlorambucil are in chronic lymphocytic leukaemia, nodular lymphomas and carcinoma of the ovary.

Melphalan (L-phenylalanine mustard, Alkeran). This mustard derivative of the amino-acid phenylalanine (Fig. 5.5) was originally synthesised with the intention that it should be effective specifically against malignant melanoma, since this amino-acid is a precursor of melanin. This specificity, however, was not achieved and the drug is no more effective against melanoma than is any other alkylating agent. Only the laevo-isomer is an active drug, but a racemic mixture is also available for use in chemo-

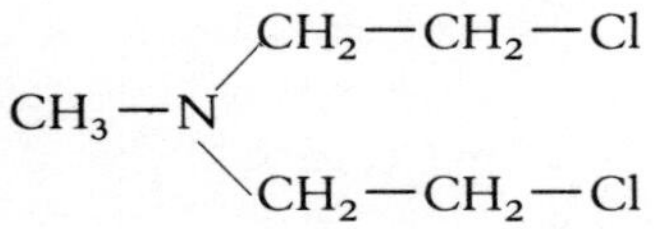

$$CH_3-N\begin{cases} CH_2-CH_2-Cl \\ CH_2-CH_2-Cl \end{cases}$$

FIG. 5.2 Nitrogen mustard.

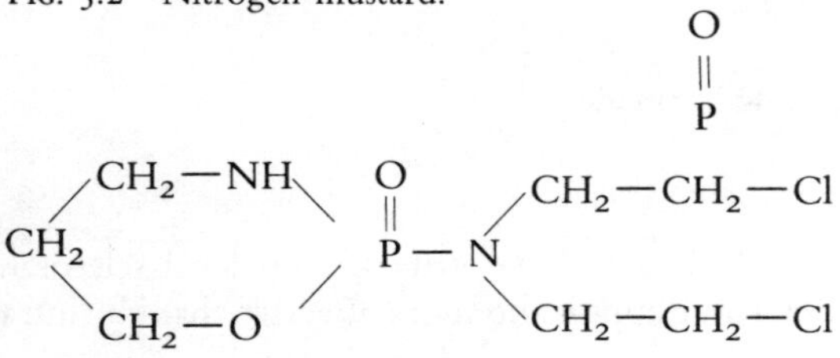

FIG. 5.3 Cyclophosphamide.

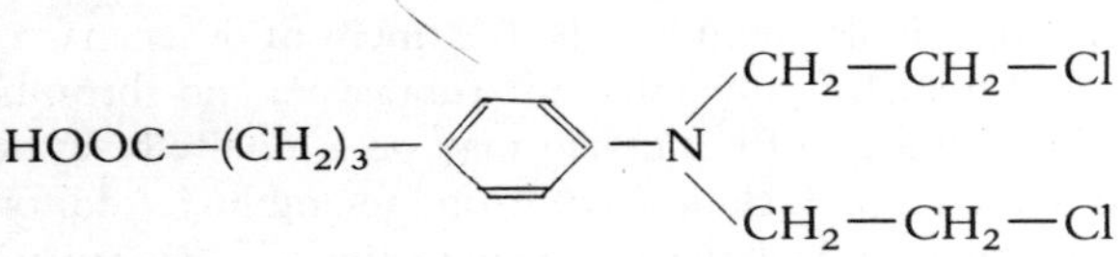

FIG. 5.4 Chlorambucil.

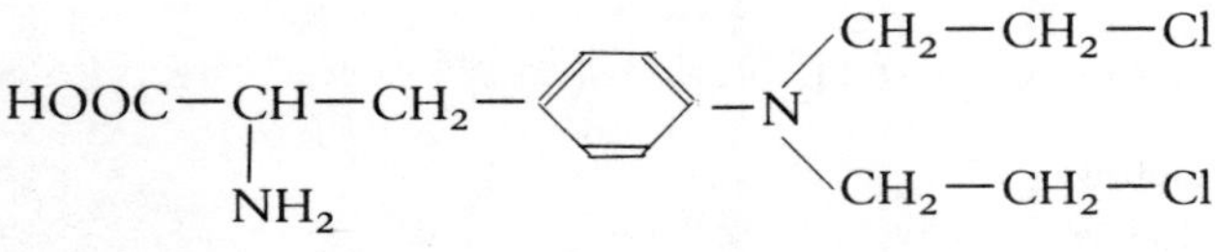

FIG. 5.5 Melphalan.

therapy known as *sarcolysin*. Melphalan is not troublesome from the point of view of side-effects, although its administration is sometimes associated with mild nausea and vomiting. Its principal use has been in the treatment of myelomatosis.

Triethylenethiophosphoramide (*Thiotepa*). This alkylating agent (Fig. 5.6), although related to nitrogen mustard, is not derived from it. It is administered parenterally and its clinical use is limited. Its major use has been in the treatment of carcinoma of the ovary, in which it is about as effective as chlorambucil, and it is also given as an intrapleural instillation in the treatment of malignant pleural effusions. This latter use, how-

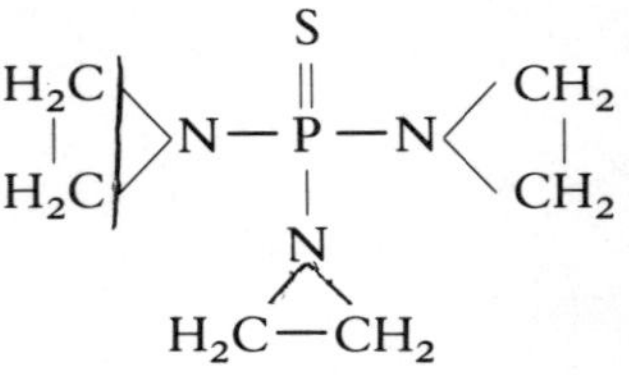

FIG. 5.6   Triethylene thiophosphoramide.

ever, is probably irrationally based as the drug has no local sclerosant action and the intrapleural route appears no more effective than the intravenous one.

Bulsulphan (Myleran). This compound, which is a methane-sulphonate, is not related chemically to the above alkylating agents (Fig. 5.7). It is well absorbed orally, has a short half-life in serum and it is excreted mainly in the urine. The principal use of busulphan is in the treatment of chronic myeloid leukaemia but it is also useful in the treatment of other marrow proliferative disorders, namely polycythaemia rubra vera and thrombocythaemia. The administration of busulphan may occasionally be associated with unusual side-effects. A clinical syndrome resembling Addison's disease occasionally occurs in which the dominant feature is skin pigmentation. Another rare side-effect is the induction of pulmonary fibrosis.

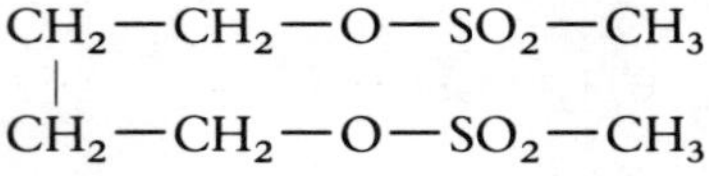

FIG. 5.7   Busulphan.

Antimetabolites

Antimetabolites interfere with various biochemical pathways, the clinically useful ones affecting DNA synthesis. The three groups of antimetabolites in clinical use are folic acid antagonists (methotrexate), antipyrimidines and antipurines.

Folic Acid Antagonists

Methotrexate (Amethopterin). The only folic acid antagonist currently in clinical use is methotrexate. Methotrexate competes with folic acid for the reductase enzyme which catalyses the conversion of folic acid to dihydrofolic acid and tetrahydrofolic acid (Fig. 5.8) and the generation of the co-enzyme, 5,10 methylene tetrahydrofolate, essential for the methylation reaction which converts deoxyuridylic acid to thymidylic

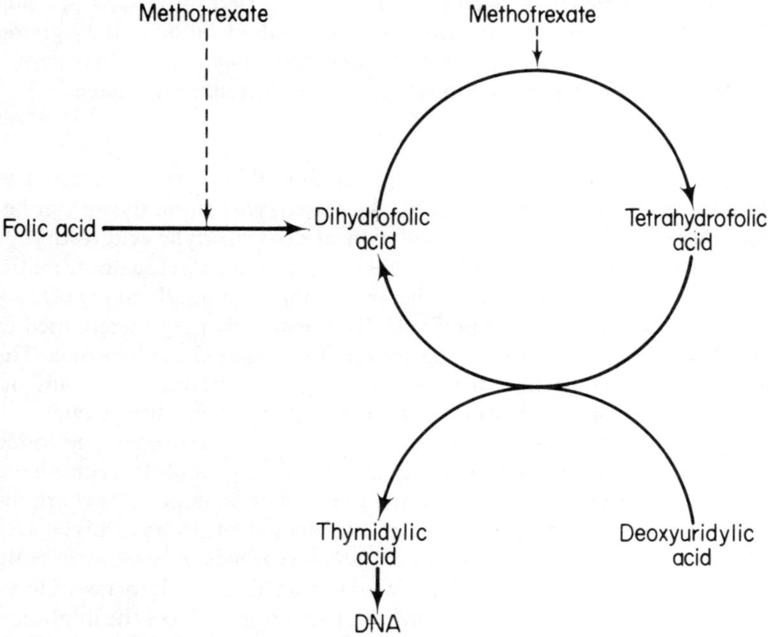

FIG. 5.8   Enzymic reactions blocked by methotrexate.

acid. In this way methotrexate interferes with the formation of DNA
so that only cells in the DNA synthetic phase (S-phase; see Chapter 1)
of the cell cycle are susceptible to this agent. Methotrexate is therefore
referred to as an *S-phase-specific agent*. As ribonucleic acid (RNA)
and protein synthesis is usually unaffected, dihydrofolic reductase production continues and DNA synthesis rapidly returns to normal after a
short exposure to methotrexate. The duration of contact of methotrexate
with the tissues, as well as the actual concentration in the blood, is, therefore, of considerable importance in determining its antimitotic effect. For
this reason, methotrexate is sometimes administered as a prolonged
infusion.

Methotrexate is excreted largely unchanged in the urine, and impairment of renal function prolongs the half-life of the drug in the body.
Renal function should therefore be assessed before this drug is used to
avoid excessive toxicity in rapidly dividing normal tissues, particularly
the bone marrow and gastro-intestinal epithelium.

Resistance to methotrexate may develop as a result of the induction
of increased dihydrofolic reductase production, or as a result of cell
membrane impermeability to the drug. Under these circumstances, resistance can be overcome using very high doses of the drug. Toxic manifesta-

tions of methotrexate can be prevented or reversed only by by-passing the reactions involved in the formation of tetrahydrofolic acid by giving the tetrahydrofolate derivative *folinic acid* (*citrovorum factor;* Leukovorin). Methotrexate has a wide spectrum of use in cancer medicine.

Antipyrimidines

5-Fluorouracil. This fluorinated pyrimidine (Fig. 5.9) is converted to fluorodeoxyuridylic acid which blocks the enzyme thymidylate synthetase, thereby inhibiting the methylation of deoxyuridylic acid to thymidylic acid and impairing DNA synthesis. 5-fluorouracil is usually administered intravenously but can also be given orally, although absorption by that route is variable and unreliable. The drug is largely metabolised in the liver, a small quantity being excreted unchanged in the urine. The major side-effect of this drug is on the gastro-intestinal tract and its principal use is in the treatment of gastro-intestinal and breast cancer.

Cytosine arabinoside (*cytarabine; Cytosar*). This is a synthetic nucleoside formed from cytosine and the sugar arabinoside (Fig. 5.9). It is considered here as an antipyrimidine because as a pyrimidine analogue it was originally thought to act by preventing the formation of deoxycytidylic acid from cytidylic acid, thereby inhibiting DNA synthesis. It has subsequently been shown that it probably acts by inhibiting DNA polymerase. However, whatever is the exact mechanism of action it involves the inhibition of DNA synthesis. It is deaminated in the liver and the metabolite excreted. The principal use of cytosine arabinoside is in the treatment of acute myeloblastic leukaemia.

Antipurines

These agents interfere with various stages in the biosynthesis of purine nucleotides but the details of their mechanism of action and metabolism are less well-known than for other antimetabolite drugs. The most commonly used antipurine is *6-mercaptopurine* (Fig. 5.10) which is used in the treatment of acute leukaemias. *Azathioprine* is the imidazolyl derivative of 6-mercaptopurine (Fig. 5.10). This drug is not commonly used as an anti-cancer agent but as an immunosuppressant, particularly in the inhibition of rejection of renal allografts. 6-mercaptopurine and azathioprine are both metabolised by the enzyme xanthine oxidase and so their actions are potentiated by allopurinol. The other antipurine in clinical use is *6-thioguanine* (Fig. 5.11) also used in the treatment of acute leukaemia; it is not metabolised by xanthine oxidase and its action is unaffected by allopurinol.

Vinca alkaloids

These drugs are naturally occurring plant alkaloids obtained from the periwinkle. They arrest metaphase in dividing cells by binding to the microtubular proteins necessary for mitotic spindle formation. In this

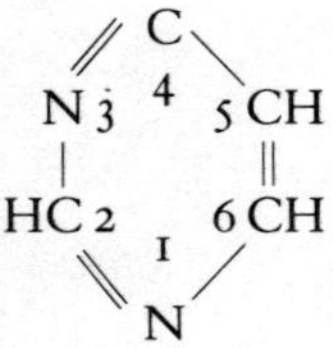

Pyrimidine

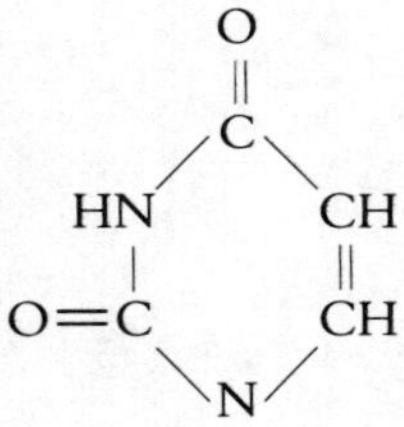

Uracil

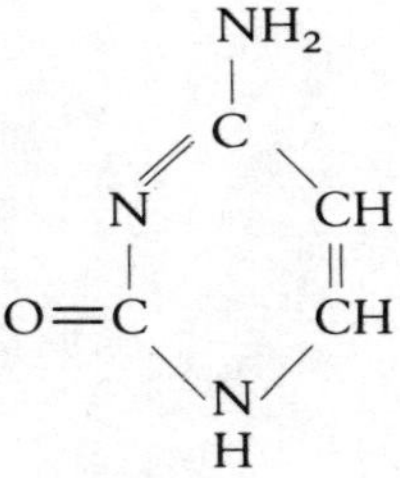

Cytosine

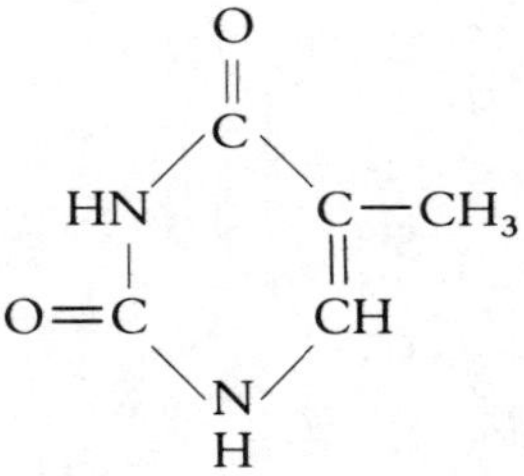

Thymine

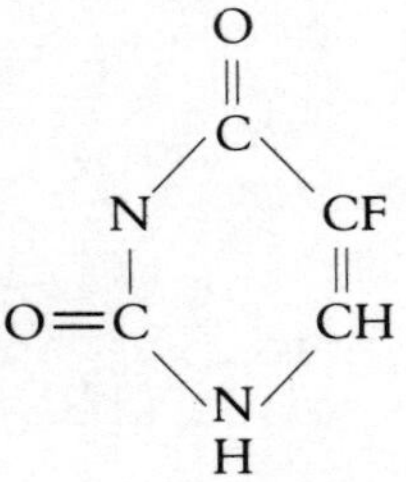

5-Fluorouracil

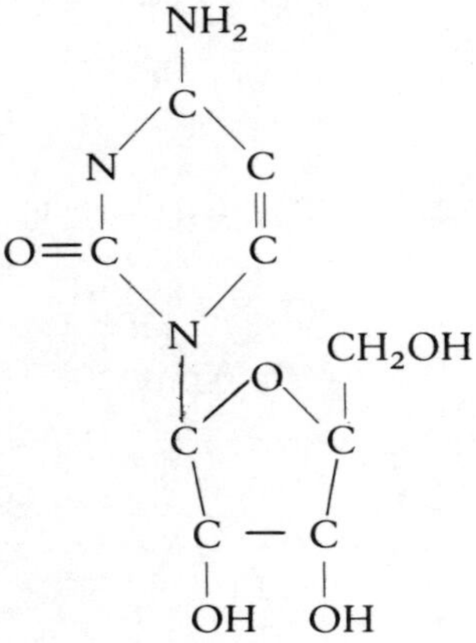

Cytosine arabinoside

FIG. 5.9 The basic pyrimidine structure, normal pyrimidine bases in DNA and RNA (uracil, cytosine, thymine) and cytotoxic pyrimidine analogues (5-fluorouracil cytosine arabinoside).

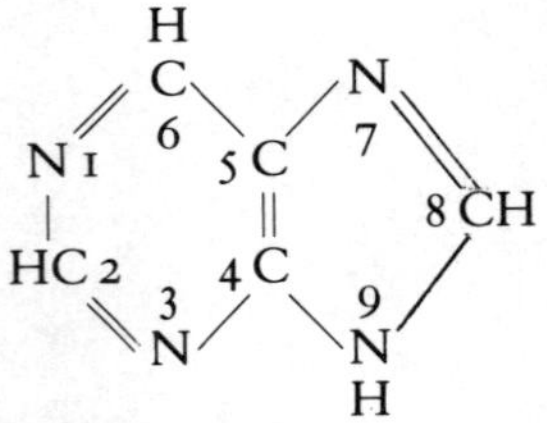

Purine

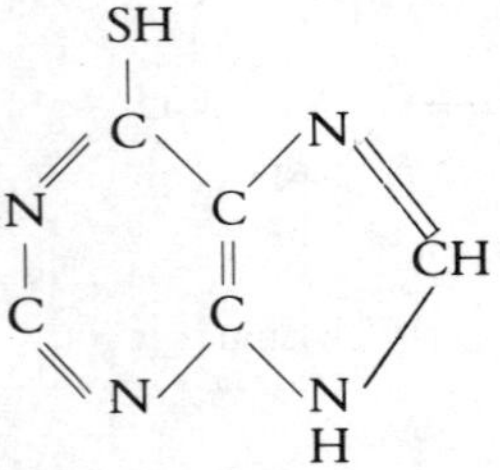

6-mercaptopurine

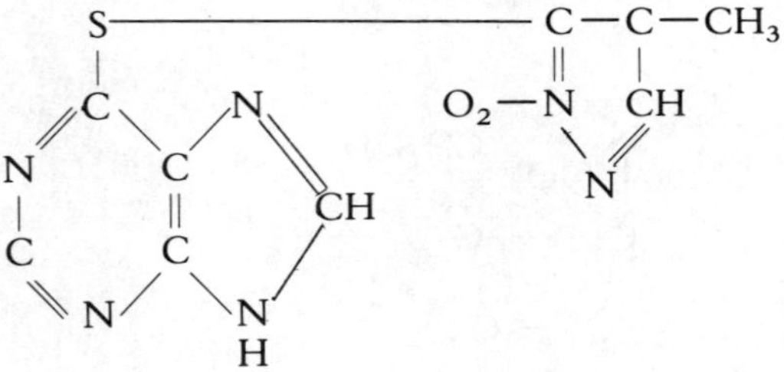

Azathioprine

FIG. 5.10 The basic purine structure and the cytotoxic derivatives 6-mercapto-purine and azathioprine.

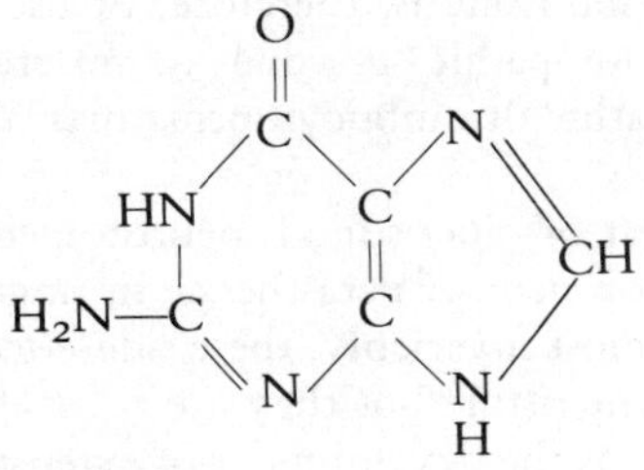

Guanine

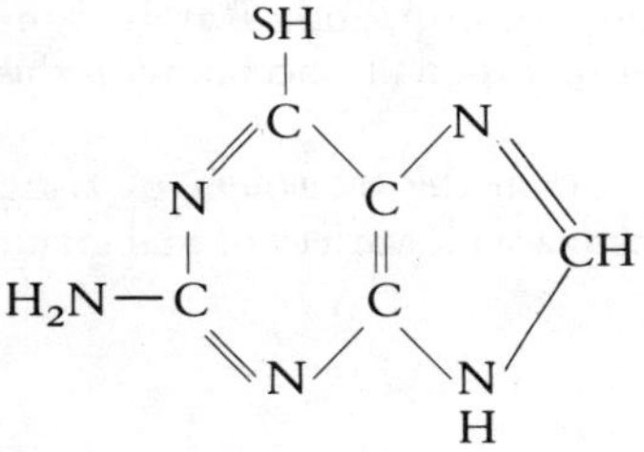

SH

6-thioguanine

FIG. 5.11   The normal purine base, guanine and its cytotoxic derivative 6-thio-guanine.

respect they are similar to the drug colchicine. They also inhibit the linkage of amino-acids to transfer RNA. These drugs are given by intravenous injection and extravasation subcutaneously causes a severe inflammatory reaction at the injection site. They are excreted by the liver into the bile. The two vinca alkaloids in clinical use are vinblastine and vincristine. Although their chemical structure is very similar they have a different spectrum of therapeutic use, different toxic effects and there is no cross-resistance between them.

Vinblastine (Velbe). Like most other cytotoxic drugs the principal side-effect is myelosuppression. This drug has a wide spectrum of clinical use, but its main use has been in the treatment of Hodgkin's disease and testicular teratomas.

Vincristine (Oncovin). This cytotoxic drug is unusual in that it has no serious toxic effect on the bone marrow. On the contrary, this drug has a stimulating effect on megakaryocytes. This effect may be attributable to a disrupting action on microtubular proteins in megakaryocytes, favouring the liberation of platelets. Vincristine is, therefore, of use in treating thrombocytopenia whether idiopathic or due to marrow destruction. Its beneficial effect in idiopathic thrombocytopenia may also be due to immunosuppression.

The important unwanted toxic effect of vincristine is neurotoxicity. This is usually manifested by the development of parasthesiae in fingers and toes and loss of tendon reflexes. Almost invariably, these side-effects eventually occur in patients receiving vincristine but they are reversible after stopping the drug. More important is the development of extensive peripheral neuropathy and the development of motor weakness necessitating the discontinuation of the drug. Other neurotoxic effects may occur. These include neuritic pain, particularly jaw pain, extra-ocular paresis, vocal cord paralysis, gait disturbances and constipation. Rarely convulsions or coma may occur. Alopecia also occasionally occurs with this drug.

The most important use of vincristine is in the treatment of acute lymphoblastic leukaemia, but it is also used in a wide variety of malignant diseases, particularly lymphomas.

Antibiotics

All the antitumour antibiotics described here are isolated from various species of Streptomyces and their interactions with DNA are responsible for their anticancer activity.

Actinomycin D (dactinomycin). This drug binds to DNA in the presence of guanine bases and inhibits RNA synthesis by RNA polymerase. It is given parenterally as it is poorly absorbed by the oral route. The half-life in the serum is short, with 50 per cent of the drug being excreted unchanged in the bile and a further 10 per cent in the urine. Careful intravenous injection is needed in order to avoid subcutaneous inflammatory reactions. Nausea and vomiting frequently occur after injection. The drug often increases the susceptibility of the skin to radiation damage and it can also cause acneiform eruptions in the absence of radiotherapy. The principal use of actinomycin D is in the treatment of embryonal tumours.

Mithramycin. This has a similar mechanism of action to actinomycin D. Its administration is also associated with nausea and vomiting but it does not cause vesicant reactions nor does it sensitise the skin to radiotherapy. This drug is useful in the treatment of testicular teratomas and apart from its antitumour effect it is capable of lowering the serum calcium which makes it of occasional use in the management of hypercalcaemia (Chapter 21).

Daunorubicin (rubidomycin, daunomycin). This drug acts by intercalating between base pairs of DNA and inhibiting RNA synthesis. It is a vesicant substance which must be given by careful intravenous injection. Its administration is associated with nausea, vomiting and the development of alopecia. An unusual toxic effect of this drug is its ability to cause myocardial damage. Acute, but transient, rhythm disturbances can occur shortly after administration, but the more serious effect is the development of a cardiomyopathy. Cardiac failure resulting from this is extremely resistant to conventional anti-cardiac failure therapy. As this effect results from a cumulative dose, it is predictable and can normally be avoided if the maximum permissible dose is not exceeded. Prior mediastinal irradiation reduces the cardiac tolerance to this drug. Daunorubicin is excreted mainly in the bile, and its toxicity is potentiated considerably if there is liver dysfunction. The principal use of daunorubicin is in the treatment of acute myeloblastic leukaemia.

Doxorubicin (hydroxydaunomycin, Adriamycin). This drug is the hydroxyl derivative of daunorubicin and it possesses a similar spectrum of toxic effects. Although doxorubicin differs very little chemically from daunorubicin it has acquired a much wider spectrum of use in the treatment of malignant tumours, particularly lymphomas, sarcomas and breast cancer.

Bleomycin. Bleomycin is the name given to a group of antibiotics which are believed to act by causing breaks in single-stranded DNA. Bleomycin has some unusual effects. Unlike other anti-tumour antibiotics it is only minimally myelo-suppressive, but its administration is often associated with the occurrence of fevers and skin rashes. The most serious toxic effect is the induction of pulmonary fibrosis, the first sign of which is the development of fine crepitations at the lung bases. This occurs before pulmonary fibrosis becomes evident radiologically and administration of the drug should be stopped before this occurs. The pulmonary toxicity is a cumulative effect of the drug and the usual maximum dose is 200–300 mg. Bleomycin has found particular use in the treatment of lymphomas and squamous cell carcinomas. This applies particularly in the head and neck region.

Mitomycin C. This antibiotic is believed to act by alkylating both DNA and RNA. It is therefore able to cross-link double-stranded DNA. It is a highly vesicant substance and has a wide range of anticancer activity.

Miscellaneous anticancer drugs

Corticosteroids

Corticosteroid drugs are widely used in the treatment of cancer. Their principal physiological actions are in the metabolism of carbohydrate, protein, fat and electrolytes, but in pharmacological doses they are able to interfere with DNA synthesis and so inhibit cell division. Lymphocytes are particularly sensitive to this effect. The toxic effects of these drugs are well-known, but these are seldom troublesome in anticancer therapy. They include the induction of Cushing's syndrome, gastro-intestinal bleeding, diabetes mellitus, psychoses and osteoporosis.

Corticosteroids are effective specifically as antitumour agents in the leukaemias, lymphomas and breast cancer. They are also of considerable use in the treatment of certain complications of cancer, particularly hypercalcaemia, thrombocytopenia, haemolytic anaemia and raised intracranial pressure.

Procarbazine. Procarbazine is a methylhydrazine derivative which causes fragmentation of DNA and interferes with DNA and RNA synthesis. Metabolites are excreted in the urine. The principal clinical use of this drug is in the treatment of Hodgkin's disease.

Hydroxyurea (Hydrea). This drug inhibits the enzyme ribonucleoside-diphosphate reductase and so interferes with the conversion of cytidylic acid to deoxycytidilic acid. It is absorbed orally and reaches a peak blood level in 2 hours. 80 per cent of the drug is excreted unchanged in the urine. This compound has been given in the treatment of chronic myeloid leukaemia and other tumours but is not now used extensively.

Dacarbazine (Dimethyl-triazino-imidazole carboxamide, DTIC). This is a new drug whose exact mode of action is unknown, although it is believed to act as an alkylating agent. Its major use clinically is in the treatment of malignant melanoma, but it is also useful in the treatment of lymphomas and sarcomas.

Nitrosoureas. The first member of this group of compounds to be introduced into anticancer treatment was *bis-chloro-ethyl nitrosourea (BCNU;* carmustine). This compound has two chlorethyl arms and probably acts as a bifunctional alkylating agent. The more recently introduced nitrosoureas, cyclohexyl-chloroethyl nitrosourea (*CCNU;* lomustine) and *methyl-CCNU* (semustine), possess one chloroethyl arm and could act as monofunctional alkylating agents. They also possess a cyclohexyl group which is able to participate in carbamylation reactions. BCNU has to be administered intravenously but CCNU and methyl-CCNU are absorbed after oral administration. Like the majority of cytotoxic drugs, the nitrosoureas suppress bone marrow, and this effect is delayed and may be prolonged, occurring six or more weeks after a single dose.

The nitrosoureas have a wide spectrum of anticancer activity but are particularly active in Hodgkin's disease. They are lipid soluble and are therefore able to cross the 'blood–brain barrier'. This led to their use in the treatment of primary and secondary intracerebral tumours. Another nitrosourea *streptozotocin* is useful in the treatment of islet-cell tumours of the pancreas.

L-asparaginase. Unlike normal cells, many malignant cells are unable to produce asparagine and are dependent on circulating asparagine for this amino-acid. L-asparaginase is an enzyme which destroys asparagine and it was hoped that it would act specifically against tumour-cell populations by depriving them of an essential amino acid which normal cells can produce. Although this drug was intended to exploit biochemical differences between normal and malignant cells, rather than kinetic differences, it has not proved particularly useful and is only occasionally used in the treatment of acute leukaemias. This agent, being a protein, is not effective after oral administration and it is almost completely metabolised. It may provoke hypersensitivity reactions.

Therapeutic strategy in cancer chemotherapy

As stated earlier, most cytotoxic drugs are toxic to all proliferating cells, but tumour cells are generally more susceptible to these agents because of the characteristics of their kinetics of growth. Cytotoxic drugs were originally administered as single agents in low dosages, often continuously, until toxicity became evident. More recently, it has become apparent that better results can often be achieved by using multiple drugs in combination given in high doses intermittently. The best results may be attained when doses approach the safe limits of toxicity. The usual toxic effect which restricts dosage is bone-marrow suppression, but certain drugs have dose-limiting effects on other tissues. For example, cardiotoxicity limits the maximum cumulative dose of adriamycin, while neurotoxicity and pulmonary toxicity limit the use of the non-myelosuppressive drugs vincristine and bleomycin respectively.

After a single dose of a marrow-suppressive cytotoxic drug has been given in the treatment of a chemosensitive tumour, cells are killed both in the tumour and in the bone marrow. However, bone marrow contains a large proportion of non-dividing stem cells which can be recruited rapidly into active cell proliferation after dividing cells in the marrow have been depleted. For this reason, recovery of bone-marrow cells is usually more rapid than in the tumour. When marrow recovery has occurred a further dose of chemotherapy can then be given with safety.

Tumour cells follow laws of *first order of kinetics*, namely that in response to a single dose of a cytotoxic agent a fixed proportion, rather than a fixed number, of tumour cells are killed. For example, if 1×10^{11} tumour cells are present and one dose of treatment kills 99 per cent of cells, then after one treatment 1×10^{9} cells will be left. If recovery allows growth to 1×10^{10} cells and a further course of treatment is then given, 1×10^{8} cells will remain and so on. These considerations are illustrated graphically in Fig. 5.12. If the proportion of cells killed by each course of chemotherapy were known then it would be possible to plan accurately the number of courses needed to eradicate completely all the tumour cells in the body. Unfortunately, this is not the case in clinical oncology except for one rare malignancy. This is *choriocarcinoma* which has the unique property of producing a specific molecule which can be detected as an excretory product in the urine, *chorionic gonadotrophin*. The amount of chorionic gonadotrophin excreted in the urine reflects the number of choriocarcinoma cells in the body. It is possible to detect the excretion of chorionic gonadotrophin when as few as one million cells are present. Treatment can then be monitored and continued until it is estimated that

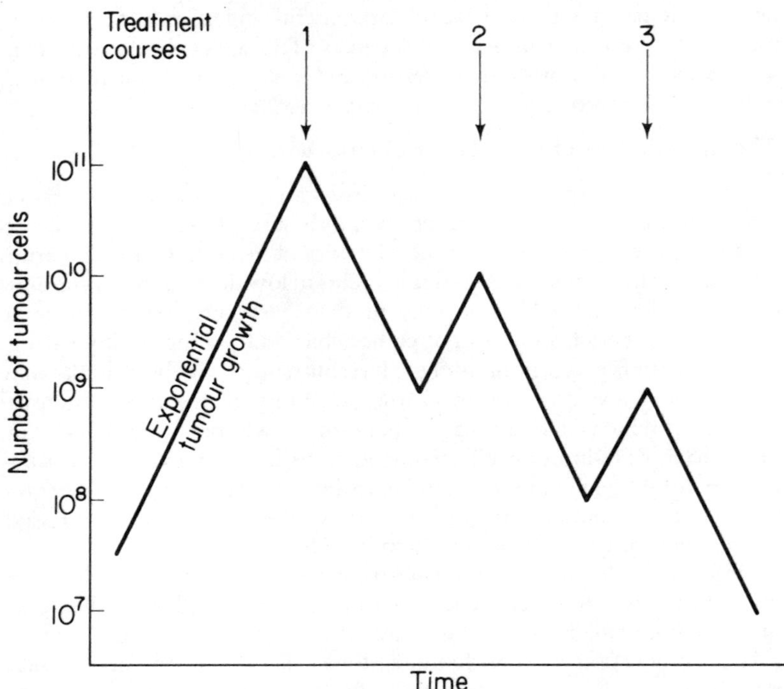

FIG. 5.12 Illustration of the sequential reduction of tumour cell by repeated courses of chemotherapy (see text).

all tumour cells have been destroyed and, by testing for this urinary hormone, recurrence can be detected at an early stage when the disease is still curable. It is this property that has, in large measure, been responsible for the curability of choriocarcinoma by chemotherapy.

Combination Chemotherapy

The rationale for giving multiple cytotoxic drugs in combination is to achieve additive killing of tumour cells. The criteria for including drugs together in combinations are as follows:

(1) each drug should be active as a single agent;
(2) each drug should affect different biochemical pathways;
(3) as far as possible the drugs should have different toxic effects.

Drug combinations with these features have high antitumour activity without additive toxicity and, because more biochemical pathways are attacked than if a single agent alone were used, there is less chance of clones of resistant cells emerging.

An example of one of the most successful drug combinations has been in the treatment of Hodgkin's disease. The combination comprises the four drugs mustine, vincristine (Oncovin), procarbazine and prednisone and is given the acronym MOPP (Fig. 5.13). This combination includes two myelosuppressive drugs (mustine and procarbazine), one which is neurotoxic (vincristine) and prednisone which has little toxicity in this combination. Each of the drugs in the combination has different mechanisms of action. The MOPP combination is far superior to any of the agents in the combination when used singly (Table 5.1) and it has made an important advance in cancer medicine by increasing the curability of Hodgkin's disease.

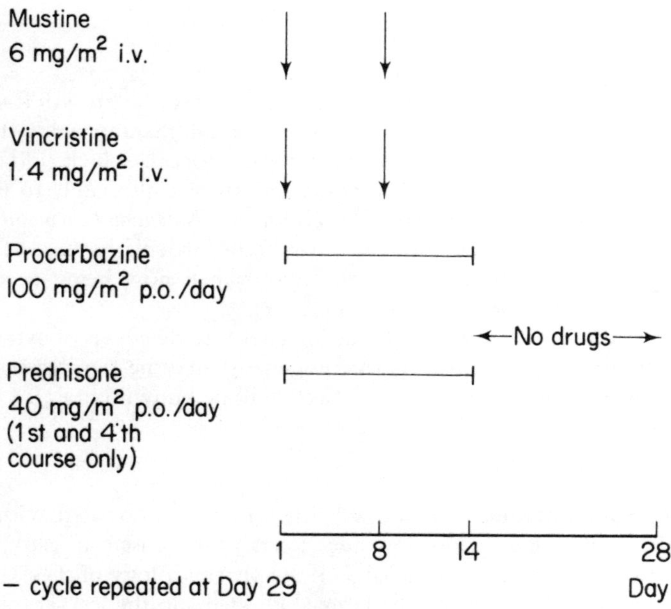

FIG. 5.13 Scheduling of drug administration in the MOPP regimen for advanced Hodgkin's disease.

'Adjuvant' Chemotherapy

Traditionally, in the treatment of cancer, chemotherapy has been reserved until local treatment has failed to control the disease and it has become advanced and disseminated. This, however, presents a situation which is intrinsically resistant to chemotherapeutic agents, because as a tumour increases in size, the proportion of cells in it undergoing division

TABLE 5.1   Remission Induction in Hodgkin's Disease by Components of the MOPP Regimen Used Singly

Treatment	Complete remissions
Mustine	13%
Vincristine	36%
Procarbazine	38%
Prednisone	0
MOPP	81%

(*Source* A. Clarysse, Y. Kenis and G. Mathé, *Cancer Chemotherapy*, Springer-Verlag, Berlin, 1976.)

decreases. In other words, as tumour size increases so the growth fraction decreases (see p. 28). It is for this reason that chemotherapy is now being employed earlier in the treatment of those cancers, which, although presenting initially as localised tumours, are known ultimately to metastasise in the majority of patients. This is known as *adjuvant chemotherapy*. The use of adjuvant chemotherapy has been particularly successful in treating embryonal tumours and this approach is now being tested in the treatment of the more common cancers.

With adjuvant chemotherapy the long-term toxic effects of cytotoxic drugs (infertility and, possibly, carcinogenesis) may be significant. The relevance and importance of these effects will be known only after long follow-up in clinical trials.

Prophylaxis against Toxicity

The administration of cytotoxic drugs may be associated with unpleasant or even life-threatening side-effects (summarised in Table 5.2). However, with adequate knowledge of the pharmacology of these drugs, all the serious side-effects can be largely avoided and the less serious but unpleasant ones prevented.

Perhaps the most common unwanted subjective side-effect is *nausea and vomiting* after the administration of many of these drugs. There is a great deal of individual variation amongst patients as to the occurrence of this effect, but for certain drugs, particularly mustine, cyclophosphamide in high doses, and certain anti-tumour antibodies, this toxic effect should be anticipated and patients given prophylactic anti-emetic therapy. Usually premedication with chlorpromazine 25–50 mg either orally or intramuscularly helps to control this. Occasionally, nausea and vomiting may be of such severe degree that admission to hospital overnight for treatment may be necessary; this is particularly so with mustine.

TABLE 5.2 Principal Side-Effects or Sites of Toxicity of Cytotoxic Drugs

Drug	Bone marrow	Nausea and Vomiting	Gut	Alopecia	Lung	Heart	Liver	Skin	Vesicant	Nervous system	Kidney	Urinary bladder	Allergy/fever
Mustine	+	+		+					+				
Cyclophosphamide	+	+	+	+								+	
Chlorambucil	+												
Melphalan	+												
Busulphan	+				+								
Methotrexate	+		+		+		+				+		
5-fluorouracil	+		+										
Cystosine arabinoside	+		+										
6-mercaptopurine	+		+				+						
6-thioguanine	+												
Vinblastine	+								+				
Vincristine				+					+				
Actinomycin D	+	+	+	+					+				
Mithramycin	+	+											
Daunorubicin	+	+	+	+		+			+				
Doxorubicin	+	+	+	+		+			+				
Bleomycin		+		+	+			+					+
Mitomycin C	+	+							+				
Procarbazine	+	+											
Dacarbazine	+	+											
Carmustine	+	+							+				
Lomustine	+	+											
L-asparginase							+						+

The toxic effects on normal proliferating tissues include *bone-marrow suppression*, loss of alimentary tract epithelium (particularly *stomatitis*) and *alopecia*. When patients have adequate doses of myelo-suppressive cytotoxic drugs leukopenia and/or thrombocytopenia occur invariably. Indeed, if these effects did not occur the adequacy of drug dosage would be in question. A knowledge of the body's handling of the drug and, particularly, the individual time courses of marrow suppression caused by the different drugs, should avoid the occurrence of potentially serious marrow suppression. Nadir white-cell counts of $2 \times 10^9/l$ and platelet counts of $70 \times 10^9/l$ are quite safe. Severe *stomatitis* has subsequently to be prevented by a decrease in the drug dosage. *Alopecia* is the one side-effect which is not preventable, and its occurrence must be anticipated and discussed with the patient before treatment is started. Its temporary nature should be explained and a wig made available for use before it is needed.

Modifications to drug dosages may have to be made in the face of abnormally functioning organs. Marrow failure may necessitate decreases in dosages while drugs normally largely excreted by the liver, for example doxorubicin, may lead to excessive toxicity if there is pre-existing liver dysfunction. In this situation appropriate reduction in dosages should be made. Drugs predominantly excreted unchanged by the kidneys, for example methotrexate, lead to excessive toxicity if there is impairment of renal function.

When it is known that toxicity may occur after cumulative administration of a drug, the relevant toxic effects should be anticipated. The occurrence of *cardiotoxicity* with daunorubicin and doxorubicin has an incidence of about 30 per cent after a predictable cumulative dose has been reached. It is expedient when using this drug to plan to give treatment to a maximum dose and then continue with alternative drugs. Bleomycin causes *pulmonary fibrosis* after a certain cumulative dose has been administered, but this can be avoided if the drug is stopped at the first appearance of crepitations at the lung bases.

Certain cytotoxic drugs interact with non-cytotoxic drugs. For example, trimethoprim-containing antibiotics may enhance methotrexate toxicity, while 6-mercaptopurine, which is potentiated by allopurinol, also causes impairment of the anticoagulant effect of warfarin. A knowledge of such drug interactions is necessary for their optimal and safe use.

The future

Future advances in the cancer chemotherapy are likely to follow:

(1) improved scheduling of agents currently in use;
(2) the development of more effective agents;
(3) the development of techniques to improve the specificity of agents, for example by exploiting antigenic peculiarities of tumour cells;
(4) the development of precise ways of monitoring response to treatment, as is now possible in choriocarcinoma;
(5) the use of drugs in early rather than in advanced disease, if necessary as an adjunct to surgery and/or radiotherapy.

PART 2

THE MALIGNANT DISEASES

CHAPTER SIX

THORAX

Metastases are among the most common tumours found in the thorax, but this chapter is concerned only with primary tumours of the lung, pleura and mediastinum.

BRONCHUS

Carcinoma

Carcinoma of the lung is synonymous with carcinoma of the bronchus from which in reality these tumours nearly always arise. There are now more than 33 000 deaths each year from lung cancer in England and Wales and the mortality has increased steadily over the last 50 years. There are four male deaths for each female death. There is considerable geographical variation although worldwide it is a very common form of cancer, especially in Europe and North America. The highest incidence is in the United Kingdom, followed by Finland and Austria.

Aetiology

There is a striking correlation between the number of cigarettes smoked daily and the death rate from lung cancer. The overwhelming evidence which indicates a relationship between cigarette smoking and this tumour is underlined by prospective studies which have revealed a reduction in the incidence of lung cancer where there has been a decrease in cigarette smoking. Recent research has shown that some patients with lung cancer have a genetically determined pre-disposition to the inducibility of the enzyme aryl hydrocarbon hydroxylase. This enzyme transforms polycyclic aromatic hydrocarbons in cigarette smoke to reactive intermediates which are carcinogenic. Other aetiological factors are to some extent masked by the effect of smoking, but they include atmospheric pollution, since lung cancer mortality is higher in urban populations than in rural communities. There are also occupational hazards which are fairly clear cut although numerically relatively unimportant. Workers with chromates, nickel, arsenic and asbestos have an increased risk of developing lung cancer. There is evidence to suggest that there may be a synergistic effect between asbestos exposure and smoking.

Pathology

The principal histological types of bronchial cancer are squamous-cell carcinoma, which is the most common, anaplastic or undifferentiated (sometimes called large-cell) in about equal proportion to oat-cell carcinoma (sometimes referred to as small-cell) and a very much smaller proportion amounting to about 10 per cent of the total are adenocarcinomas which, unlike all of the others, are not related to smoking. Rarely, tumours arise from the alveolar or bronchiolar epithelium, and are referred to as alveolar-cell carcinomas.

The great majority of bronchial carcinomas arise centrally in the main or segmental bronchi. Some begin peripherally and of these a few, usually adenocarcinomas, originate in old scar tissue. Spread occurs by direct local extension into adjacent lung or structures of the chest wall and mediastinum. Lymph nodes become involved early and spread takes place through the hilar, mediastinal, paratracheal and cervical lymph nodes. Spread in the blood also occurs early and distant metastases occur frequently in the brain, liver, adrenals and bones. Trans-bronchial spread is uncommon except in the case of alveolar cell carcinoma which may alternatively have a multicentric origin.

Bronchial carcinomas, more than any other tumour, have a remarkable capacity to produce polypeptides which have an effect similar to normally occurring hormones and give rise to non-metastatic manifestations of lung cancer (Chapter 17).

Clinical features

These depend partly upon the histological type of tumour (oat-cell carcinomas for instance are those which most frequently produce ectopic hormones), whether or not it has metastasised, and its site within the bronchial tree. A careful history is extremely important and often leads to a strong suspicion of the diagnosis, whereas physical signs may either be absent altogether or reveal definite abnormalities.

Symptoms relating to a tumour within the chest include a recent cough or a change in the character of an existing cough (remembering that many patients are smokers and therefore already have chronic bronchitis). Haemoptysis is relatively common and highly significant. Dyspnoea may be due to obstruction of a major bronchus with or without collapse of a lung or lobe, a pleural effusion or the presence of consolidation. Pain is usually due to infiltration of the pleura, chest wall or mediastinal structures. Dysphagia may be caused by compression of the oesophagus and hoarseness occurs when vocal-cord paralysis results from infiltration of the left recurrent laryngeal nerve.

Often by the time of presentation, carcinoma of the lung has already produced metastases which may cause enlarged lymph nodes in the neck, cerebral metastases with a variety of neurological abnormalities, liver involvement with nausea, anorexia, abdominal pain and jaundice or pain due to metastases in bone.

Physical signs depend on the site and type of tumour. Carcinoma of the lung commonly presents as pneumonia with the signs of either lobar, segmental or less well-defined consolidation. Collapse of a lobe may occur due to bronchial obstruction. A pleural effusion can be present which is likely to be bloodstained and tends to recur after aspiration. The signs of superior vena caval obstruction are striking and are nearly always due to a central carcinoma of the bronchus which has extended into the structures of the mediastinum. Occasionally tumours near the apex of the lung erode the first rib, the lower part of the brachial plexus, causing pain in the shoulder and arm, and, since the sympathetic pathways may be involved, an ipsilateral Horner's syndrome. These signs constitute Pancoast's syndrome. Clubbing of the fingers occurs in a proportion of patients and is sometimes accompanied by hypertrophic pulmonary osteoarthropathy.

Investigations

A chest radiograph (postero-anterior and lateral views) is the most important initial investigation for establishing the diagnosis. The solitary rounded opacity of a peripheral tumour may undergo central necrosis and then be revealed as a shaggy, thick-walled cavity. More often, however, as the tumour is central in origin, the evidence for its existence is indirect and produced by partial obstruction to a bronchus, causing atelectasis or, occasionally, localised emphysema. Impaired drainage causes infection distally with pneumonia which may be recurrent or slow to resolve. Other features include pleural effusion, elevation of the diaphragm due to pulmonary contraction, or involvement of the phrenic nerve with diaphragmatic paralysis, rib erosion and hilar or mediastinal node enlargement. Lymphatic infiltration may be seen to spread out from the hilar region peripherally into the lung. Occasionally tomography may be helpful to show a lesion or anatomical deformity in more detail. Although in the past bronchography has been valuable to indicate the nature of an obstruction to relatively small bronchi, it is seldom undertaken now.

Cytological examination of the sputum in experienced hands shows malignant cells to be present in as many as 80 per cent of patients when multiple fresh specimens are collected. The diagnosis is more likely to be established in this way with central tumours, but peripheral lesions also exfoliate cells into the bronchi, and these cells may be expectorated and identified in the sputum. The use of a flexible bronchial brush introduced selectively into peripheral bronchi through a bronchoscope enables cytological specimens to be obtained with more precision and improves the diagnostic accuracy with some peripheral lesions.

Bronchoscopy is required in the majority of patients suspected of having bronchial carcinoma in order to provide a specimen for histological proof of the diagnosis, but more particularly to determine whether the lesion may be amenable to operative treatment. The introduction of the fibre-optic bronchoscope has made it possible to examine successfully more peripheral bronchi than hitherto, particularly those in the upper lobes.

Other methods of obtaining the diagnosis include needle biopsy of a peripherally placed lesion using fluoroscopic control, but this carries a risk of producing a pneumothorax and a lesser risk of bleeding. Although it is sometimes necessary to undertake a thoracotomy in order to establish the diagnosis with certainty and to assess the feasibility of radical surgery, it is clearly undesirable to do this when the tumour has already meta-stasised. For this reason scalene node biopsy and mediastinoscopy can be undertaken when it is suspected that lymph nodes in these regions are involved or in some patients in whom the diagnosis is uncertain. These procedures yield a high incidence of positive results.

In the presence of a pleural effusion, cytological examination of the fluid often reveals malignant cells, but there may be diagnostic difficulties, particularly after pulmonary infarction. Pleural biopsy using an Abram's needle may reveal metastatic spread to the parietal pleura.

Other investigations are necessary to identify possible metastases and these may include liver-function tests and liver and bone scintiscans. It is also important to consider the patient's general condition and fitness for radical treatment. The history will reveal whether he is able to under-take physical effort without breathlessness, but it is useful to watch the patient walk and talk simultaneously to assess this capacity. Respiratory function tests will indicate more precisely the extent of any ventilatory impairment.

Treatment

Surgery offers the best prospect of long-term survival in patients who have a tumour of suitable histological type which is favourably situated and where there are no metastases. In practice this usually means patients with squamous-cell carcinomas which are localised so that lobectomy or pneumonectomy achieves complete removal. For this to be possible the patient (who will often have chronic bronchitis) must have sufficient respiratory reserve, which can normally be assessed from his exercise tolerance. Pneumonectomy should not be undertaken if the forced vital capacity is less than half the predicted value or if the arterial pCO_2 is elevated above normal. This is usually reflected by the patient being breathless on walking along the flat and having to stop. Most clinicians would recommend radical surgery for very few patients over the age of 70, although some are fit for this type of treatment.

When the tumour is an oat-cell carcinoma, even though it may be apparently operable, the overall results of surgery are so bad that it is now usual practice to recommend other forms of treatment. Radical radio-therapy is usually advised and consists of giving supervoltage irradiation to large fields. 5000 to 6000 rads in 4–6 weeks are used and this is the treatment of choice in oat-cell tumours, when surgery would otherwise be technically feasible, and in squamous and adenocarcinomas when surgery is contraindicated for other reasons. Palliative radiotherapy is used in patients with tumours considered inoperable. Such treatment may prolong survival when the disease is confined to the chest. Palliative radiotherapy is also useful to relieve superior vena caval obstruction and occlusion of large airways causing atelectasis and dyspnoea. Haemoptyses can be controlled by radiotherapy, which is also useful to treat painful metastases in the skeleton.

Oat-cell carcinoma responds to cytotoxic chemotherapy and, using combinations of drugs, regressions are seen in about 50 per cent of patients. Current effective combinations include cyclophosphamide + methotrexate + CCNU and Adriamycin + vincristine + procarbazine. The regressions achieved have a median duration of about 9–12 months. It is not yet certain that these regressions lead to an improved survival but clinical trials currently being conducted should clarify this. Non-oat-cell carcinomas of the lung are not regularly responsive to cytotoxic agents and effective combinations have not yet been determined. Alleviation of superior vena caval obstruction can be achieved by an intravenous infusion of mustine, which is usually given into a leg vein where venous flow is faster under these circumstances. In elderly patients where the tumour is inoperable, there may be no symptoms and specific treatment is therefore not required. This policy may also be adopted in younger patients when there is no prospect of cure and when treatment may lead to unpleasant symptoms without any benefit. The management of pleural effusions is discussed in Chapter 20.

Prognosis and survival

Half the patients at the time of diagnosis are not suitable for major surgery either because of the extent of disease or coexisting medical conditions. Of the remainder, half are found to have inoperable tumours at thoracotomy. Therefore, only approximately 25 per cent of patients with this disease undergo resection of the tumour and only a quarter of these are alive five years later. This gives an overall survival rate of 5 per cent. It is of interest that some patients who have had an empyema post-operatively have been among the longest survivors and this has led to the so far unsupported suggestion that post-operative infection of this kind has enhanced the immunological response to the tumour. However, work on immunological aspects of lung cancer has not proved rewarding. The appalling survival of patients with this tumour is a dismal commentary on a largely preventable disease.

Adenoma

The term bronchial adenoma is somewhat misleading and is used to describe more than one condition, which may sometimes be malignant.

The more common is the carcinoid which is found usually in a main bronchus or near the orifice of a lobar bronchus. It is a slow-growing tumour with a smooth endobronchial surface which, viewed through a bronchoscope, is round, red and may be pedunculated; ulceration does not occur. The principal symptom is usually recurrent haemoptysis which may be severe, or it may present because of the effects of bronchial obstruction with atelectasis, dyspnoea or infection. It occurs slightly more often in females than in males and is usually seen in the 20–40 age group. It may not appear on a chest radiograph, although tomography will sometimes reveal its presence, but 90 per cent are visible through the bronchoscope which is the only means of establishing the diagnosis.

The treatment is to resect the tumour, if possible, through a bronchotomy in order to preserve lung tissue. Systemic symptoms due to the production of pharmacologically active substances do occur but are unusual in this tumour, as distinct from metastatic carcinoid arising from the alimentary tract.

Another variety of so called bronchial adenoma is the cylindroma or adenoid cystic carcinoma, a malignant tumour which tends to grow very slowly over many years and has a variable prognosis. It is more invasive than the carcinoid, and if it is not resectable radiotherapy is often helpful.

PLEURA

The one pleural tumour of importance is the mesothelioma. This was first described among asbestos miners in South Africa. Since then there was first a gradual, then a steep rise in the incidence of this tumour in many parts of the world. There are now more than 200 cases annually in the United Kingdom, chiefly amongst dockyard workers and those exposed to blue asbestos (crocidolite). The latent period between exposure and development of the tumour is long, frequently 30 years, and it seems that only a relatively short exposure may be required to induce this tumour.

The presenting symptoms are pain in the chest accompanied by a pleural effusion which recurs after aspiration. The side of the chest gradually becomes fixed and pain increases. Chest radiographs show initially an effusion with increasing pleural shadowing and the development of large nodular shadows along the pleural surface. Autopsy reveals the contracted lung to be enveloped in a thick, rigid casing of tumour. Spread occurs into the mediastinal structures, distant metastases being rare.

Treatment appears to have little effect upon the course of the tumour. Radiotherapy and chemotherapy are occasionally of use. Radical resection is possible but is usually a formidable undertaking, recurrence being the rule and death inevitable.

MEDIASTINUM

Metastases in the mediastinum are common (particularly from primary tumours of the lung) and lymphomas either present or are found at this site. Carcinomas of an intrathoracic thyroid are rare and tumours of the thyroid in the neck usually produce symptoms outside the chest. The three groups of tumour which are relatively common in the mediastinum are tumours of nervous tissue, thymomas and teratomas.

Tumours of nervous tissue

Although these are considered to be the most common primary tumours originating in the mediastinal area they arise from nervous tissue in the paravertebral gutter, occur at all ages, and are usually benign, since malignant tumours occur most commonly in childhood. They arise in the intercostal nerves, the sympathetic chain and embryonic neurogenic rests. The neurofibromas and neurilemmomas are benign but may undergo malignant change to become neurosarcomas. In the case of neurofibromas, these occur either singly or in association with generalised neurofibromatosis. These may grow through an intravertebral foramen (causing its enlargement seen radiographically) giving rise to a 'dumb-bell' tumour with spinal-cord compression. Ganglioneuromas arise from the sympathetic chain and have a more marked tendency to become malignant, particularly in children. Neuroblastomas arise from sympathetic nervous tissue and occur almost exclusively in children, in whom they are highly invasive tumours.

Neurological tumours, particularly the benign ones, are usually asymptomatic and found during a routine chest radiograph. Sometimes pain is present due to root involvement and there may also be cough. Ganglioneuromas and neuroblastomas may produce catechol-amines and give rise to abdominal distension and diarrhoea or raised blood pressure and sweating and increased urinary excretion of vanilyl mandelic acid. Malignant tumours of childhood may present with dyspnoea or cough and in the case of neuroblastomas have a reasonably good prognosis in children under one year who are treated adequately by resection, followed by radiotherapy, and, if necessary, chemotherapy (Chapter 19).

Thymomas

These are the second most common of the primary mediastinal tumours, occurring in the anterior mediastinum, usually in adults.

Histologically it can be very difficult to determine whether a thymoma is benign or malignant and the decision is usually made because of the clinical and pathological behaviour of the tumour rather than its microscopic appearance. About 25 per cent of thymomas are malignant and invade the lungs, pericardium and adjacent blood vessels and lymphatics, but distant metastases are rare.

Thymomas are diagnosed either as a result of a routine chest radiograph which shows a rounded shadow in the anterior mediastinum, or because of the symptoms produced by the malignant tumour. These may be related to superior vena caval obstruction, cough and dyspnoea because of invasion of the lungs or involvement of the pericardium. A number of patients (quoted figures vary from 10 to 50 per cent) with malignant thymoma have myasthenia gravis which first suggests the presence of this tumour, and this is particularly so in men. Other endocrine abnormalities occur, such as Cushing's syndrome due to ectopic adrenocorticotrophin production, and other associated conditions such as red-cell aplasia and hypogammaglobulinaemia have also been described. Surgical resection is the usual treatment as it is necessary to establish the diagnosis and determine the extent of the tumour. Often it is not feasible to remove it completely, so that radiotherapy is also given. Malignant thymoma is particularly radio-sensitive.

Teratomas

These tumours, which occur in adults, are found in the anterior mediastinum. They are closely related embryologically to dermoid cysts which occupy the same site but which are usually considered to comprise only the ectodermal component, while teratomas contain cells from each of the three germinal layers. This distinction is incorrect since dermoid cysts, when examined microscopically, usually contain some elements from the other germinal layers and indeed may undergo malignant change. Nevertheless, dermoids are usually cystic and benign tumours whereas teratomas are solid and more frequently undergo malignant change.

These tumours are usually sharply defined rounded shadows with calcification seen on a chest radiograph. The diagnosis can only be made with certainty after surgical exploration and the treatment is resection combined, if necessary, with radiotherapy. The prognosis for malignant teratomas is poor.

CHAPTER SEVEN

ALIMENTARY SYSTEM

Malignant tumours developing in the alimentary system, most commonly in the colon and rectum, account for over half the cancers in clinical practice.

OESOPHAGUS

The majority (approximately 98 per cent) of oesophageal cancers are squamous-cell carcinomas, the remainder being adenocarcinomas.

Carcinoma

Carcinoma of the oesophagus occurs more commonly in men than women. Its incidence is higher in Scotland than elsewhere in the United Kingdom, other areas of high prevalence being Japan, China and in the vicinity of the Caspian Sea. Conditions predisposing to this cancer include achalasia of the cardia, the Plummer–Vinson syndrome, congenital short oesophagus and chronic severe peptic oesophagitis, which may, rarely, complicate hiatal herniae.

Pathology

Squamous-cell carcinoma occurs throughout the length of the oeso-phagus, adenocarcinoma occurring at the cardia. In women these tumours tend to occur in the upper half, in men the lower half. They infiltrate the oesophageal wall, fungate into the lumen and occasionally ulcerate. Stenosis and occlusion of the oesophageal lumen develops rapidly. Spread outside the oesophagus initially involves the para-oesophageal lymph nodes which spread subsequently to lymph nodes in the neck and upper abdomen. Invasion of other intrathoracic structures (especially trachea and aorta) is common and metastases to the lungs and liver occur.

Clinical features

The usual symptom of carcinoma of the oesophagus is progressive dysphagia, with hoarseness and haematemesis occurring occasionally. As oesophageal obstruction progresses, weight loss, becomes marked and aspiration of oesophageal contents may lead to pneumonitis. Invasion of the great vessels may cause massive haemorrhage producing a terminal haematemesis.

Investigations

The diagnosis of carcinoma of the oesophagus, often obvious on clinical grounds, is confirmed radiologically by a barium swallow which shows a constant narrowing of the oesophagus with irregularity of the luminal surface. Histological proof of the diagnosis should be obtained by examination of a biopsy specimen taken at endoscopy.

Treatment

The results of attempts to cure in carcinoma of the oesophagus are very poor. The overall 5-year survival rate is less than 5 per cent, but in patients suitable for surgical treatment this rises to 10 per cent. However, the surgery involved is extensive with a post-operative mortality of about 20 per cent. The usual operation to attempt cure is total oesophagectomy with either a stomach 'pull-up' procedure, anastomosing the pharynx and stomach in the upper mediastinum, or movement of a section of colon together with its mesentary to the mediastinum for anastamosis between the pharynx and stomach. Although controlled trials have not been performed, it seems that radical radiotherapy can achieve the same results as surgery with rather less morbidity.

Palliative treatment of this condition includes radiotherapy which in less than radical doses can achieve relief of dysphagia in a high proportion of patients. Later in the disease relief of dysphagia can be achieved by inserting a tube into the oesophageal lumen at the site of obstruction. Intubation procedures, however, may be complicated by haemorrhage and fistula formation, and they may become displaced or obstructed by tumour. Feeding gastrostomies have been done in the treatment of carcinoma of the oesophagus, but in many instances this is not worthwhile since it merely prolongs the terminal illness. Chemotherapy is currently of little use in this disease, although occasional regressions have been reported with alkylating agents. Bleomycin which has been shown to be effective against squamous-cell cancers has been investigated, but, used as a single agent, results have been poor and its eventual role may be in combination with other agents. The use of chemotherapy as an adjunct to surgery or radiotherapy to achieve cure of this disease has still to be investigated. In the treatment of adenocarcinomas of the cardia, as for adenocarcinomas of the stomach, chemotherapy has shown more promise (see below).

STOMACH

Several types of malignant tumours develop in the stomach, the majority (approximately 95 per cent) being adenocarcinomas; the remainder include squamous-cell carcinomas, adenoacanthomas, carcinoid tumours, lymphomas and leiomyosarcomas.

Carcinoma

Carcinoma of the stomach may be seen at any age but is most common in middle to late life, with a slightly higher incidence in males. It is the fifth most common cause of death from cancer in the West. There is a particularly high incidence of gastric cancer in Japan. The cause of adeno-carcinoma of the stomach is unknown, but pernicious anaemia is a well-established predisposing condition, and there is an increased occurrence in patients with blood group A, gastric ulcer, chronic atrophic gastritis or after partial gastrectomy.

Pathology

Adenocarcinoma may arise in any area of the stomach, but more than half of these tumours occur in the pylorus and antrum. Occasionally it has a multicentric origin. Macroscopically it may be ulcerative, polypoid, scirrhous or superficially infiltrative, while histologically it may vary from a highly cellular tumour to a predominantly fibrous one in which few tumour cells are present. There is a wide spectrum of cellular differenti-ation from a well-differentiated glandular pattern to an anaplastic appear-ance; mucin production is variable.

Gastric carcinoma may invade locally to involve the omentum, liver, pancreas, oesophagus or colon, the latter sometimes resulting in the formation of a gastro-colic fistula. Spread to regional lymph nodes in the upper abdomen and to distant lymphatic sites, particularly the left supra-clavicular fossa (Virchow's node) is common. Vascular spread to other sites, most commonly the liver, and dissemination of cells within the peritoneal cavity may also occur.

Clinical features

The most common presenting symptom of gastric carcinoma is epi-gastric discomfort. In the early stages this symptom is often relieved by belching, but eventually it becomes increasingly severe and persistent. Anorexia and weight loss are common and, as the primary tumour increases in size, nausea and vomiting develop and complete pyloric obstruction may occur. Carcinomas at the cardia cause dysphagia. Anaemia is common, and occult blood loss in the stools may be found, but both clinical haematemesis and melaena are uncommon. Rarely perforation of an ulcerating primary may lead to peritonitis.

Quite frequently emaciation may be the only feature but physical examination may show liver enlargement, palpable nodes in the left supra-clavicular fossa or nodules around the umbilicus. Carcinoma of the stomach is the malignancy most frequently associated with dermatomyo-sitis and acanthosis nigricans (see Chapter 12).

Investigations

Anaemia is usually microcytic and hypochromic due to chronic blood loss, but macrocytic if there is associated pernicious anaemia. Barium meal is the most important examination in the investigation of this tumour. The radiological changes include filling defects in the stomach lumen, distortion of its shape, ulceration, loss of distensibility and alterations in the mucosal pattern. Carcinomas situated at the cardia are often difficult to demonstrate radiologically. Occasionally it may be difficult to distinguish between a benign gastric ulcer and an ulcerating carcinoma. Gastroscopy is a valuable investigation during which a biopsy is taken to provide histological confirmation of the diagnosis, while cytology of exfoliated cells in brushings obtained at endoscopy is often positive in gastric carcinoma.

Treatment

The only potentially curative treatment for gastric cancer is surgical excision and, depending on the local extent of the disease, either sub-total or total gastrectomy is the appropriate operation. Unfortunately, at the time of laparotomy most gastric cancers are too far advanced for cure to be achieved, and the overall 5-year survival of patients is approximately 10 per cent. Survival after operation depends largely on regional lymph-node involvement, and if this has not occurred the 5-year survival is as high as 50 per cent compared with only 5 per cent when the nodes are involved. Palliative resection of the tumour or by-pass procedures are occasionally appropriate and feasible. Radiotherapy has little role in the treatment of gastric cancers except for relieving pain from localised bony metastases.

It has become apparent from recent investigations that of the common tumours arising within the alimentary system, gastric cancer is probably the most chemosensitive. For some time 5-fluorouracil was the principal drug used, and in patients with advanced disease achieves regressions in about 20 per cent, but these are of short duration. However, other agents, particularly nitrosoureas, mitomycin C and adriamycin have been shown to be effective and better results are now being obtained with these agents used in combination. Until recently chemotherapy has been reserved for treating advanced inoperable disease, but studies have now begun in which adjuvant chemotherapy as part of the primary management of resectable tumours is being investigated.

Screening

In view of the high prevalence of gastric cancer in Japan, screening programmes employing radiological and endoscopic techniques have been established. There is some evidence to indicate that this approach can lead to the earlier detection of this disease and an associated higher cure rate.

However, gastric cancer remains a major cause of death in Japan. At the present time, because of low cost effectiveness, such screening programmes are not feasible in countries where the disease is less common.

SMALL INTESTINE

Despite its length and enormous mucosal surface area, the small intestine is only occasionally the site of malignant disease. The most common neoplasms are carcinoid tumours, but adenocarcinomas, lymphomas and leiomyosarcomas also occur.

Carcinoid tumours

These small, round-celled argentaffin-positive tumours probably arise from the Kulchitsky cells in the crypts of Lieberkühn. Frequently small in size, they may remain asymptomatic during life, being discovered only at autopsy. Carcinoid tumours have a similar incidence in both sexes. The most common site of origin is in the ileum, the majority being situated in the terminal part, but they also occur in the oesophagus, stomach, duodenum, bile ducts, pancreas, Meckel's diverticulum, appendix, colon, rectum, ovary, testes, larynx and bronchus. Occasionally they appear to have a multicentric origin.

Although usually of small size, the primary growth may be large enough to give rise to abdominal pain, intestinal obstruction, diarrhoea, weight loss and, rarely, intestinal bleeding. Carcinoid tumours have an extremely slow growth rate and tendency to disseminate. They may be locally invasive involving the peritoneum and mesentery or distant metastases may occur, particularly in the liver and lungs. Occasionally, metastatic carcinoid tumours give rise to the carcinoid syndrome (see below).

The curative treatment for carcinoid tumours is surgical excision, the 5-year survival rate being 90 per cent, but even inoperable tumours may be associated with long survival (40 per cent at 5 years). These tumours are resistant to radiotherapy but a variety of chemotherapeutic agents (including cyclophosphamide, melphalan, actinomycin-D, 5-fluorouracil and streptozotocin) may induce short-term regressions. However, in view of the indolent course of these tumours chemotherapy is usually not indicated. Cytotoxic drugs must be used with great caution in the presence of the carcinoid syndrome (see below).

Carcinoid syndrome

Occasionally carcinoid tumours produce high levels of the pharmacologically active substances 5-hydroxytryptamine, kinins, catecholamines, histamine and prostaglandins which lead to the appearance of the carcinoid syndrome. The features of this striking clinical syndrome occur virtually exclusively in the presence of hepatic metastases. They include cutaneous flushing, bronchoconstriction, hypotension, oedema and intestinal hypermotility causing diarrhoea. Development of fibrous plaques on the endo-cardium of the right side of the heart leads to the development of pul-monary stenosis and tricuspid incompetence; rarely left-sided cardiac lesions may occur. The pathogenesis of carcinoid heart disease is not under-stood.

The diagnosis of carcinoid syndrome is sometimes obvious from the clinical features, but certain investigations are usually necessary for its con-firmation. Measurement of 5-hydroxyindoleacetic acid in the urine is often helpful, while chromatography of the urine may show the presence of other metabolites of 5-hydroxytryptamine. A provocation test with intra-venous noradrenaline to induce flushing may be performed cautiously and is often diagnostic. Other assays are available to determine the presence of other pharmacologically active substances in urine and plasma.

Although symptoms due to the presence of the primary carcinoid tumours are treated by resection, the carcinoid syndrome may require specific pharmacological treatment. Flushing is difficult to treat success-fully but responds to alpha-receptor blockage with phenoxybenzamine. Alpha-methyl-dopa, corticosteroids, phenothiazines or cycloheptadine may all be useful, while diarrhoea and bronchospasm should be relieved by methysergide. Treatment of cardiac failure may be required. Occasion-ally effective relief of the carcinoid syndrome is achieved by surgical resection of large metastatic deposits.

The chemotherapeutic agents mentioned above as sometimes being effective for primary carcinoid tumours may also be used to treat the syndrome. They should be used with great care and in lower doses, since, if the tumour is particularly chemo-sensitive, its disintegration may precipitate a severe carcinoid crisis and death.

APPENDIX

Neoplasms of the appendix are rare. Adenocarcinoma may present as acute appendicitis, intestinal bleeding or rarely intussusception and the appropriate treatment is right hemicolectomy. Occasionally adeno-carcinomas of the appendix are mucin-secreting and give rise to pseudo-myxoma peritonei. This condition has a protracted course and long sur-vival is usual. Carcinoid tumours of the appendix are usually benign but rarely may metastasise and give rise to the carcinoid syndrome.

LARGE INTESTINE

Cancers of the colon and rectum together form the most common group of malignant diseases in Europe and North America. As causes of death from cancer, colo-rectal tumours are surpassed only by carcinoma of the breast in women and carcinoma of the bronchus in men. 98 per cent of colo-rectal tumours are adenocarcinomas, the remainder comprising squamous-cell carcinomas, carcinoid tumours, lymphomas and leiomyosarcomas.

Adenocarcinoma

The overall incidence of adenocarcinoma of the large intestine is about the same in both sexes, but there is a slightly higher preponderance of colonic tumours in women, while rectal tumours are slightly more common in men. The disease is rare before the age of 40 but thereafter the incidence rapidly increases with age. The incidence increases in migrants from areas of low incidence to areas of high incidence, suggesting that large-bowel cancer is environment-related. There has been much speculation on the possible factors involved, such as fats, proteins and low fibre content of the diet, the last of which may influence intestinal transit time, but conclusive evidence of a definite association has not yet been forthcoming. There are, however, conditions which clearly pre-dispose to adenocarcinoma of the large bowel, namely familial polyposis coli and ulcerative colitis. Villous adenomas probably also give rise to invasive cancer, as do large (>2 cm diameter) adenomatous polyps.

Pathology

Large-bowel carcinomas are predominantly distal in distribution, about 40 per cent occurring in the rectum, 20 per cent in the sigmoid and 11 per cent in the descending colon. The sites of the remainder in order of decreasing frequency are caecum, ascending colon, transverse colon, splenic flexure and hepatic flexure. Anatomically, these tumours usually form well-defined intraluminal masses with overlying ulceration; less commonly, diffuse infiltrating tumours occur. Rectal carcinomas may be friable and papillary in form. Occasionally large-bowel cancers appear to have a multicentric origin and this is usually associated with pre-existing polyposis coli or ulcerative colitis. Histologically, these tumours vary in differentiation from well-defined neoplasms, closely resembling normal mucosa, to highly anaplastic tumours bearing no such similarity.

Large-bowel cancers spread circumferentially in the bowel wall, eventually resulting in obstruction. Direct invasion may involve adjacent organs including stomach, duodenum, liver, pancreas, small bowel, kidney, spleen and abdominal wall for colonic tumours, or bladder, prostate, ureters, vagina, sacrum and sacral plexus for rectal tumours. Spread to regional lymph nodes is common, with tumours in the colon meta-stasising to mesenteric and para-aortic nodes, while rectal tumours spread to nodes in the groin, pelvis and then to the para-aortic region. Spread up the thoracic duct may lead to involvement of supraclavicular lymph nodes. Vascular spread results in metastases to the liver, lungs, and, less commonly, bones, brain, adrenal glands and kidneys. The spread of large-bowel cancer is commonly expressed in Duke's classification:

Type A   tumour confined to the mucosa and submucosa;
Type B   invasion through the muscularis without nodal metastasis;
Type C   involvement of regional lymph nodes.

This classification correlates well with survival; the five-year survival for type A being about 70 per cent, type B 45 per cent and type C 20 per cent.

Clinical features

Frequently, the first symptoms of carcinoma of the large bowel, a minor change in bowel habit or vague abdominal discomfort, are often ignored for a long time and the average duration of symptoms in this disease at the time of presentation is about 12 months. More specific symptoms of large-bowel cancer depend upon the site of the tumour. Because of the fluid consistency of proximal colon contents, tumours at this site grow to a relatively large size before causing obstruction, and these tumours are generally associated with increasing abdominal discomfort, diarrhoea and weight loss, while chronic occult blood loss leads to anaemia. In the left side of the colon, where the bowel contents are more solid and the lumen small, obstruction occurs earlier with tumours of smaller size, and constipation associated with spasmodic abdominal pain is a common complaint. Rectal cancers are associated with increased frequency and urgency of defaecation, tenesmus and passage of mucus and frank blood is more common than with more proximal tumours. Pain is unusual with rectal tumours unless invasion of extra-rectal pelvic structures has occurred. The physical signs of carcinoma of the large bowel are variable. The primary tumour may be palpable, and, depending on the stage of the disease, there may be features of cachexia and anaemia. Lymphatic spread may lead to enlargement of nodes in the groins or supraclavicular fossae. Hepatomegaly and jaundice indicate metastases in the liver and ascites may be present. Digital examination of the rectum discloses the presence of the majority of rectal cancers.

Investigations

Haematological and biochemical investigations may show the presence of anaemia, impairment of liver function, or renal failure from ureteric obstruction. The presence of occult blood in the stools is common and exfoliative cytology has been found to be useful in a few centres, but this technique is not used widely.

Sigmoidoscopy is an important examination and, in view of the predominant distal distribution of these tumours, about 60 per cent can be discovered by this technique. More recently, fibre-optic endoscopy of the colon has been introduced, and this allows the whole colon to be visualised. The majority of large-bowel cancers can be demonstrated radiologically using contrast media containing barium. For the best results to be obtained, this investigation should be preceded by preparing the bowel with laxatives and enemas. Definition of lesions can be sharpened by double-contrast studies using air and barium. The characteristic finding, radiologically, is a consistent filling defect at the site of the tumour. Intravenous urography may demonstrate the presence of ureteric obstruction.

In 1965, the discovery of carcinoembryonic antigen (CEA) in patients with tumours of the colon engendered optimism that such tumours could be diagnosed early by the detection of this substance. Unfortunately, this hope has not been realised and further studies have shown CEA to lack specificity. It can often be demonstrated in association with other tumours, particularly of the lung, pancreas, stomach, liver, breast, prostate and ovary, and also with several benign conditions including ulcerative colitis, benign colonic polyps, cirrhosis of the liver, pancreatitis, chronic renal disease and chronic obstructive airways disease. It is probable that the ultimate value of estimating CEA will be in monitoring a patient's progress after removal of a tumour, when a subsequent increase in the plasma level may be an early indication of impending relapse.

Treatment

The curative treatment for carcinoma of the large bowel is surgical resection of the primary tumour with a wide margin of normal bowel on each side, together with the regional lymph nodes in continuity.

The usual operation is a right or left hemicolectomy depending on the site of the tumour. For proximally situated rectal tumours an anterior resection with colo-rectal anastamosis can be performed, but for distal rectal tumours an abdomino-perineal resection of the rectum with permanent colostomy is necessary. The results of surgical treatment for operable tumours depend upon Duke's classification as mentioned previously. Some preparation before operation to clear the bowel of as much of its contents as possible is needed, but attempts to sterilise the bowel flora are unnecessary and may predispose to staphylococcal enterocolitis.

Primary inoperable tumours, or locally recurrent tumours, can be palliated effectively by radiotherapy. Chemotherapy has been generally disappointing in large-bowel cancer, although 5-fluorouracil has been used extensively. Because of different criteria adopted by investigators for including patients in studies and for assessing results, response rates varying between 8 and 85 per cent have been reported for this drug. These have been of short duration, only exceptionally lasting more than a few months. It is probable that with combination chemotherapy the situation will improve and suitable drugs include 5-fluorouracil, mitomycin C, nitrosoureas (particularly BCNU and MeCCNU) and vincristine. The place of radiotherapy and chemotherapy in conjunction with surgery for the primary treatment of localised disease is currently being investigated.

Because of the high risk of carcinoma developing in patients with ulcerative colitis, much attention has been given to prophylactic colectomy in these patients. Probably over one third of patients with ulcerative colitis would eventually develop carcinoma and the incidence increases the longer the disease has been present. In ulcerative colitis, carcinoma has a particularly poor prognosis; the tumours are often anaplastic and the 5-year survival after surgical resection is about 15 per cent. There is general agreement that ulcerative colitis of long standing should be treated by total colectomy, but whether the rectum too should be removed, with a permanent ileostomy, or ileo-rectal anastamosis performed, is controversial. The rectum after ileo-rectal anastamosis remains a likely site of carcinoma, but protagonists of this approach suggest that frequent proctoscopic examinations would detect this at an early stage when removal of the rectum could then be undertaken. It is the safety of this latter approach which has been questioned.

Cancer of the large bowel eventually develops in nearly all patients with polyposis coli. This disease is inherited as a Mendelian autosomal dominant but also occurs as a result of gene mutation. Prophylactic colectomy is always considered in this disease, but the extent of colectomy to be advised here has also been the subject of debate. It is probable that only in that minority of patients without involvement of the rectum by polypoid disease is it safe to leave the rectum, but in all other cases total colectomy with removal of the rectum and ileostomy is probably the correct preventative procedure. Alternatively, the rectum may be left intact, provided regular proctoscopic examinations are performed with electrocoagulation of polyps.

ANUS

Though a variety of malignant diseases (including basal-cell carcinomas, Paget's disease, Bowen's disease and melanoma) occur in the anus, over 90 per cent of primary cancers in this region are squamous-cell carcinomas. Tumours of the anus are relatively uncommon, being thirty times less frequent than in the adjacent rectum. These tumours present as either nodules, ulcers, indurated areas or polypoid masses. Local invasion of the perianal tissues occurs and lymphatic spread may cause enlargement of inguinal lymph nodes which is occasionally the first clinical manifestation. Venous invasion leads to distant metastases usually in the liver, lungs and bones. The most common symptom is bleeding while many patients experience anal discomfort or pain and advance of the tumour eventually leads to interference with defaecation.

Well-differentiated small anal cancers are often successfully treated by local excision but for more advanced tumours abdominoperineal resection is necessary. Should involvement of inguinal lymph nodes become apparent after surgical resection of the primary tumour, a second operation to dissect the groin may improve the prognosis, but when the nodes are clinically involved at the time of first presentation this procedure does not benefit the patient as more disseminated metastases are invariably present. In patients unsuitable for surgery, radiotherapy is sometimes curative, but this form of treatment is more frequently used for palliation. Adequate information on the use of chemotherapy in this disease is not available.

LIVER

In Europe and North America, the usual tumours to affect the liver are metastases from primary sites elsewhere, particularly those in the gastro-intestinal tract. The most common primary liver tumour is the hepatoma (hepatocellular carcinoma) accounting for about 90 per cent of primary liver cancer. Cholangiocarcinomas form most of the remaining primary liver tumours, others being exceedingly rare but include haemangio-endothelioma, Küpffer cell sarcoma, hepatoblastoma, which occurs exclusively in childhood (Chapter 19) and miscellaneous sarcomas. In certain Eastern and African countries, primary liver cancers are more common, and in some regions they are the most frequently occurring abdominal cancer.

Hepatoma

Many chemical carcinogens, notably dimethylbenzanthracine, cause experimental tumours in laboratory animals, but no clear association has been demonstrated between these compounds and human hepatomas. One substance, however, which has been considered aetiologically important is aflatoxin, which is produced in peanuts infected by a species of Aspergillus, and there is some suggestion that kwashiorkor may predispose to hepatomas. An increased incidence of hepatocellular carcinoma occurs in patients with cirrhosis of the liver, particularly haemochromatosis.

Most hepatomas have a nodular pattern throughout the liver, but they may also be diffuse or form large single masses, and cellular differentiation is highly variable. Invasion of surrounding structures is unusual, but these tumours commonly infiltrate the portal and hepatic veins. In the latter case, extension may occur up the inferior vena cava, even as far as the right atrium. Hepatomas are vascular tumours and haemorrhage into the peritoneal cavity may occur. In about one third of cases, distant metastases develop, particularly in the regional lymph nodes and lungs.

Rare before the age of 40, the incidence of hepatomas increases thereafter and these tumours are more common in men. With pre-existing cirrhosis, recognition of a hepatoma is difficult, but is suggested by an exacerbation of symptoms (increasing jaundice, hepatomegaly, ascites, epigastric pain and cachexia). For tumours arising in a non-cirrhoic liver, the usual symptom is upper abdominal pain, but less commonly they may present with intraperitoneal haemorrhage, an enlarging mass in the upper abdomen, or jaundice due to obstruction of the bile ducts. Non-metastatic manifestations of hepatoma include hypercalcaemia, hypo-glycaemia, polycythaemia, gynaecomastia and cutaneous porphyria. Bio-chemical tests show derangement of liver function if there is co-existing cirrhosis, but are frequently normal in its absence. A chest radiograph frequently shows elevation of the right dome of the diaphragm and an isotopic liver scan usually delineates the tumour. Such scans may be of considerable value in directing the site of a percutaneous liver biopsy to acquire tissue for histological diagnosis. A biopsy is usually diagnostic for well-differentiated tumours but with anaplastic lesions it may not be possible to differentiate between primary liver cancer and metastases from other sites. However, the finding of an embryonic protein, alpha feto protein, is usually confirmatory for a primary hepatoma, as the only other diseases consistently showing elevated levels of this substance are embryonal tumours and malignant testicular teratomas. The prognosis for hepatomas is poor, and the five-year survival is almost nil. Although tumours may be technically resectable such procedures do not appear to increase survival. Total hepatectomy with liver transplantation is being investigated in some centres. Radiotherapy has not proved of value for palliation, but short remissions may be obtained occasionally with chemo-therapy using 5-fluorouracil and BCNU.

Cholangiocarcinoma

These tumours usually arise from intrahepatic bile ducts and histo-logically are similar to those arising in extra-hepatic bile ducts. Their occurrence is not related to pre-existing cirrhosis, but an important pre-disposing factor is infestation by the liver fluke Clonorchis sinensis. The clinical features and prognosis are similar to those of hepatoma.

GALL BLADDER

Carcinoma of the gall bladder is about three times more common in women than men and there is considerable evidence suggesting an aetio-logical association with cholelithiasis, sclerosing cholangitis and ulcerative colitis. These tumours are adenocarcinomas with varying degrees of dif-ferentiation. Early spread is to regional lymph nodes and direct extension to the liver is common. Local complications include empyema of the gall bladder, acute cholecystitis, haemorrhage, obstructive jaundice, pyloric and duodenal obstruction and the formation of fistulae with other hollow viscera. Blood-borne spread through the hepatic and portal veins occurs and distant metastases are seen most frequently in the peritoneum, ovaries, pleurae and lungs.

The most frequent presenting symptom of carcinoma of the gall bladder is right hypochondrial pain, often radiating to the back, and a mass is usually palpable in the right hypochondrium with sometimes an overlying rub heard on auscultation. Anorexia, nausea, vomiting, weight loss, jaundice and ascites are common.

Oral cholecystography usually fails to demonstrate the gall bladder, but on occasion a filling defect within the organ is seen. Obstruction of the cystic duct may be seen with intravenous cholangiography and chest radiography often shows a small right-sided pleural effusion and sometimes elevation of the right hemidiaphragm.

Over 80 per cent of gall-bladder cancers are unresectable at laparotomy, but biliary diversion may be technically feasible and useful for palliation. Radiotherapy has proved of little value, and there is no adequate information on the use of chemotherapy. Despite the possible association between this tumour and cholelithiasis, there seems little justification to recommend prophylactic cholecystectomy on these grounds for the not uncommon finding of asymptomatic gall stones. The median survival of patients with carcinoma of the gall bladder after diagnosis is less than three months.

EXTRA HEPATIC BILE DUCTS

Carcinoma developing in the extrahepatic bile ducts are rare, more so than carcinoma of the gall bladder. Like cholangiocarcinoma there appears to be an aetiological relationship to *Clonorchis sinensis* infestation. Bile-duct cancers spread along the ducts and may invade the adjacent pancreas, liver, duodenum, portal vein and hepatic artery. The usual clinical feature is progressive jaundice, most patients having pruritus. Upper abdominal pain is present in about half the patients and there is often weight loss, nausea, anorexia and, sometimes, fever due to cholangitis. Hepatomegaly is common and, if the disease is prolonged, cutaneous xanthomas appear. Biochemical investigations confirm the presence of obstructive jaundice. Intravenous cholangiography is of little use for localising the tumour, which usually awaits laparotomy, but pre-operative percutaneous transhepatic cholangiography may be valuable in planning surgery. If this is precluded because of bleeding problems then endoscopic retrograde cholangiography should be considered.

Rarely is this tumour curable, but tumours situated in the middle of the common bile duct can sometimes be completely resected and end-to-end anastomosis performed. Occasionally, radical pancreaticoduodenectomy may be curative for distal tumours. Usually, however, only palliation by insertion of a T-tube can be achieved by surgery. Bile-duct cancers are usually radio-resistant and chemotherapy with 5-fluorouracil produces only occasional regressions, invariably of short duration. Death usually occurs from hepatic failure or cholangitis.

AMPULLA OF VATER

Because of its anatomical site, carcinoma of the ampulla becomes clinically apparent at an early stage, when it produces obstructive and sometimes fluctuating jaundice, liver enlargement and dilation of bile ducts and gall bladder. This tumour spreads relatively slowly, at first involving local structures (common bile duct, second part of the duodenum and head of pancreas), and later, the splenic and portal veins and liver. Associated symptoms include upper abdominal pain, pruritus, weight loss, fever from cholangitis and occult blood loss leading to anaemia.

Ampullary carcinoma may be diagnosed on a barium meal and by endoscopic examination at which a biopsy, or specimen for duodenal cytology, can be taken.

Because this tumour is often small when detected, surgical excision may be curative; the 5-year survival rate after pancreaticoduodenectomy is as high as 40 per cent. For unresectable tumours, cholecystoduodenostomy is a useful palliative procedure. Radiotherapy has not been of value and there is little information on the use of chemotherapy.

EXOCRINE PANCREAS

The great majority of cancers of the exocrine pancreas are adenocarcinomas; other tumours being exceedingly rare, 75 per cent of carcinomas occur in the head and are usually firm scirrhous tumours with surrounding pancreatitis. Carcinoma of the pancreas is increasing in importance as a cause of death and is usually advanced at the time of diagnosis. Direct invasion of the adjacent duodenum, stomach, colon, kidney and inferior vena cava occur and metastases in the liver are common, but also occur in the peritoneum, lungs, bone and adrenal glands. Males are more commonly affected than females and there is an increasing incidence of the disease with age.

Pain is the common presenting feature and is characteristically vague and poorly localised; it may be felt in the abdomen or back. Carcinoma of the head of the pancreas leads to obstructive jaundice and, sometimes, steatorrhoea due to obstruction to flow of pancreatic secretions. Weight loss is common and diabetes mellitus occurs in 10–20 per cent of patients; thrombophlebitis migrans is an occasional association. On examination jaundice and hepatomegaly may be present, but physical signs are often lacking in this disease.

A barium meal may demonstrate abnormalities in the appearance of the duodenum suggesting the presence of a pancreatic growth and selective angiography or scanning after the injection of radioactive selenium-labelled methionine may also assist in diagnosis. Endoscopic retrograde examination of the common bile and pancreatic ducts, which is becoming more widely used, is helpful. Grey-scale ultrasonography and CT scanning are likely to be used more in the future.

The diagnosis, however, usually awaits confirmation at laparotomy, which shows the tumour to be unresectable in most cases. When the tumour is situated in the head of the pancreas, about one quarter of cases are suitable for radical excision. This is done by Whipple's operation at which the head of the pancreas, duodenum and pylorus are excised and pancreaticojejunostomy, choledochojejunostomy and gastrojejunostomy are performed. The operative mortality of this operation is high (about 20 per cent) and the most encouraging figures shows a 5-year survival rate after this procedure of about 15 per cent. Usually, surgery has to be palliative and diversion of bile, by choledochojejunostomy and gastro-enterostomy may give the patients considerable relief. However, after these procedures, the median survival is only 4 or 5 months, but this is longer than if no palliative procedure at all is performed. Radiotherapy alone has little to offer for the palliation of this disease and responses to chemotherapy are infrequent and short-lived. The drug with which the most experience has been gained is 5-fluorouracil, but the addition of a nitrosourea (BCNU) appears to increase the effectiveness of chemo-therapy. More encouraging results have been achieved recently by com-bining radiotherapy with chemotherapy.

Symptomatic and supportive therapy in carcinoma of the pancreas are important and include the control of diabetes mellitus, correction of steatorrhoea, by the administration of pancreatic enzymes, fat restriction or dietary adjustment (for example substituting medium-chain tri-glycerides, which do not require lipase digestion for absorption, for other fats), and relief of pruritus by administering cholestyramine or phenothia-zines.

ENDOCRINE PANCREAS

Tumours of the islets of Langerhans are rare, but their occurrence is associated with well-defined clinical syndromes. Islet-cell tumours remain relatively small and are often benign; local invasion and distant metastases are rare. These tumours may occur in ectopic pancreatic tissue and in 10–15 per cent of cases they are multiple.

Insulinoma

The most common functional islet-cell tumour is the insulinoma which, in 90 per cent of cases, is a benign adenoma, the remainder showing characteristics of malignancy. This tumour gives rise to recurrent episodes of hypoglycaemia aggravated by fasting and due to the excessive insulin production. During the attack very low levels of sugar occur and rapid reversal of symptoms is achieved by administering intravenous glucose. A tolbutamide tolerance test may also be helpful. This produces a profound and persistent hypoglycaemia associated with high insulin levels.

Insulinomas should be treated by excision but at laparotomy a tumour is not always apparent on exploration of the pancreas. In these circum-stances, blind resection of the pancreas is carried out in progressive steps, from the head to the tail, with intra-operative monitoring of the blood sugar; occasionally total pancreatectomy is required. For malignant, non-resectable insulinomas, a high remission rate can be obtained with strepto-zotocin.

Zollinger–Ellison syndrome

Gastrin-secreting tumours of the pancreas, usually carcinomas, result in the production of large amounts of gastric acid. This syndrome is characterised by recurrent peptic ulcers which are often multiple. Diarrhoea is a feature of this syndrome, probably caused by the inactivation of pancreatic lipase by excess acidity. High basal gastric acid secretion is almost diagnostic of this condition and a barium meal demonstrates hypertrophy of the gastric rugae and a rapid intestinal transit time. High serum gastrin levels can be detected by a radioimmunoassay.

The appropriate treatment is resection of the gastrin-producing tumour, but if this is not possible, useful palliation of the symptoms can be obtained by total gastrectomy.

Pancreatic cholera

Recently a syndrome of profuse, watery diarrhoea, hypokalaemia and hypochlorhydria (pancreatic cholera) associated with an islet-cell tumour has been described. The clinical features are probably attributable to high levels of vaso-active intestinal peptide (VIP) produced by the tumour. Resection is often curative but, if this is not possible, streptozotocin is effective in inducing remissions.

Alpha-cell tumour

Alpha-cell tumours, characterised by the production of large quantities of glucagon with consequent hyperglycaemia, have been described but are excessively rare.

PERITONEUM

The peritoneum is frequently a site of metastases from tumours elsewhere characterised clinically by the production of ascites. The only tumour arising primarily in the peritoneum is mesothelioma.

Mesothelioma

Mesiotheliomas arising in the peritoneum are rare, being less common than those developing in the pleura (Chapter 6), but like the pleural tumours are also associated with prior asbestos exposure. Mesotheliomas may be distributed throughout the peritoneum as nodules or may form a single large tumour mass. This tumour spreads by direct invasion, particularly of the diaphragm, and metastasis is rare. The usual presenting symptom is pain, weight loss is common, ascites usually present and bowel obstruction may occur.

At diagnosis these tumours are usually unresectable, and radiotherapy and chemotherapy have not been shown to have any palliative value. Treatment, therefore, comprises analgesia and paracenteses to relieve abdominal distension. Survival is rarely more than a year from diagnosis.

CHAPTER EIGHT

BREAST

The term breast cancer is used synonymously with carcinoma of the breast. Other malignant tumours, including metastases from primary tumours elsewhere, also occur in the breast but these are much less common and are not considered in this chapter.

CARCINOMA OF THE BREAST

This is the most common malignant tumour of women in the West. It has protean clinical manifestations and is illustrative of all types of cancer therapy. A study of carcinoma of the breast, therefore, provides a broad survey of the principles of clinical oncology.

Epidemiology

The incidence of this disease in the United Kingdom is about 70 cases per 100 000 of the female population per annum, and nearly 12 000 women die of this disease each year. Predominantly a disease of the female sex, the incidence in the male is some 100–200 times less. The worldwide incidence of this disease is very variable. While it is the most common malignant tumour of women in the West, it is relatively rare in the Orient. The reason for these differences in the incidence are not understood, but they are probably environmental rather than genetic (see Chapter 2).

Aetiology

Although the cause of human breast cancer is unknown, several factors increasing the risk of the disease in an individual by 2–5 fold can be identified. These include close family history of the disease, late first pregnancy, previous benign disease, nulliparity and low urinary androgen excretion.

In laboratory mice, mammary carcinomas can be induced by the ingestion of dimethylbenzanthracine. Another murine mammary tumour is induced by a virus known as the Bittner milk factor which is transmitted from generation to generation during lactation. So far no chemical or viral cause has been demonstrated conclusively for human breast cancer.

Pathology

Carcinomas arise from the epithelium lining the lactiferous ducts or alveoli of the breast. These tumours can vary from highly cellular carcinomas, with little stromal content, to fibrous masses containing relatively few malignant carcinoma cells (scirrhous carcinomas). The histopathological features can be graded according to the degree of glandular differentiation, cell pleomorphism and the nuclear appearances. Generally, the less well-differentiated the tumour and the higher the mitotic activity, the poorer the prognosis. Occasionally breast carcinomas appear to arise from multiple sites within the breast. The primary tumours are locally invasive and metastasise to the regional lymph nodes in the axilla, internal mammary chain and supraclavicular fossa, and by the blood to distant sites. The most common site of distant metastases is bone, particularly the spine, pelvis and ribs. Other common sites of dissemination are the skin and subcutaneous tissues, lungs, pleurae, liver, peritoneum, ovaries and brain.

Clinical features

Breast cancer usually presents as a painless lump in the breast, when it has to be differentiated from other breast lumps, particularly benign cysts, areas of fibroadenosis and fibroadenomata. Local signs assist in the differential diagnosis: deep fixation of the lump or palpable regional lymph nodes favour the diagnosis of carcinoma.

Skin attachment and dimpling should be noted and involvement of the skin by carcinoma is indicated by overlying cutaneous oedema (peau d'orange), thickening of the overlying skin, infiltration, frank eruption of the primary tumour through the skin (fungation), skin ulceration or surrounding satellite skin nodules.

Immobility of the breast lump over deep structures indicates fixation to the chest wall. If movement of a mobile lump is decreased with pectoraalis major muscle contracted then fixation to this muscle or its fascia can be inferred.

Enlarged lymph nodes may be palpable in the axilla and supraclavicular fossa, and occasionally enlarged internal mammary nodes may be evident protruding parasternally through the intercostal spaces. Should axillary nodes be palpable then it is necessary, for subsequent management, to note whether the nodes are discrete and freely mobile or whether they are matted to each other or adherent to skin or deep structures. Palpable discrete lymph nodes in the axilla may be normal or they may show reactive hyperplasia or contain metastatic cancer. Clinical assessment is incorrect in about 30 per cent of cases and axillary dissection is necessary to quantify accurately the degree of axillary-node involvement. The importance of this in management is discussed below.

Occasionally breast cancer may present as Paget's disease of the nipple. This condition appears as a moist eczema which may progress to ulceration. There is always an underlying breast carcinoma. Rarely the first clinical sign of breast cancer is a nipple discharge which may contain occult or macroscopic blood, but in most cases this occurrence is due to a benign intraduct papilloma.

The presenting features of breast cancer may be due to distant metastatic disease. This is particularly seen with skeletal metastases when the first evidence of disease may be bone pain or a pathological fracture. Occasionally, the presenting feature may be dyspnoea due to the presence of a pleural effusion, but presentation of breast cancer due to metastases in other sites is rare.

The clinical features of metastatic disease are dependent upon the sites of the lesions. Commoner manifestations include pleural effusions, bone deposits, when spinal collapse may result in spinal cord compression, hepatic dysfunction, hypercalcaemia and marrow suppression.

Investigations

To distinguish carcinoma from benign or other malignant tumours of the breast, the diagnosis must be confirmed by histological examination of a biopsy specimen. Normally, an excision or incision biopsy of the primary tumour or, alternatively, a biopsy of one of the regional lymph nodes can be performed. We prefer an elective biopsy to confirm the diagnosis of carcinoma before further investigation and treatment, but an alternative approach is the examination of a frozen section specimen at operation and to proceed with a more extensive operation under the same anaesthetic. However, this latter approach does not permit further elective investigations, nor does it give the clinician an opportunity to discuss the planned management with the patient after the diagnosis is known for certain.

In the case of a nipple discharge, where no underlying mass is palpable, it is necessary to identify the duct from which the discharge arises. This is then explored surgically (microdochectomy) which usually uncovers an intraduct papilloma. When Paget's disease is suspected, this diagnosis is confirmed by histological examination of a nipple biopsy.

When the diagnosis of carcinoma has been confirmed, further investigations should be done in order to assess the spread of the tumour. This enables definition of the stage of the disease on which subsequent treatment will be based. A full blood count should be done and a blood film examined. A decrease in any of the formed elements or a leucoerythroblastic blood picture suggests marrow involvement by the tumour. This may be confirmed by examination of a marrow aspirate or biopsy. Biochemical tests should be done to exclude any metabolic disorders, particularly disturbances of liver function or the presence of hypercalcaemia. A chest radiograph and radiographs of the skull, spine, pelvis and femora (skeletal survey) should be done to search for pulmonary, pleural or skeletal metastases. Alternatively, the skeleton can be assessed by isotopic bone scanning with radiography of areas of increased uptake. These tests should be regarded as essential in all cases and occasionally other selected tests will be appropriate in individual cases, for example, brain and liver scans.

Staging

After full clinical assessment and investigations, the extent of all clinically detectable disease should have been determined and this can be expressed in terms of staging. The stage of the disease is of immediate importance in deciding the most appropriate treatment. The staging system given here is simple and practical and differs only in detail from the TNM classification (Chapter 3).

Stage 1. The primary tumour is confined to breast tissue. There may be attachment to the skin but not frank involvement, nor is there any attachment to deep structures. There is no detectable spread to regional lymph nodes, nor evidence of distant metastases.

Stage 2. The primary tumour has the same characteristics as Stage 1 but there is spread to ipsilateral axillary lymph nodes which remain discrete and free from attachment to skin, or deep structures or each other. There is no detectable spread to other lymph nodes, nor are there distant metastases.

Stage 3. This is locally advanced disease without distant metastases. One or more of the following features determines this staging:

   (1) involvement of the skin as shown by:
      (a) peau d'orange
      (b) skin infiltration
      (c) skin ulceration
      (d) fungation
      (e) satellite skin nodules
   (2) attachment of the primary tumour to deep structures
   (3) ipsilateral axillary nodes fixed to one another or to skin or deep structures
   (4) involvement of supraclavicular or infraclavicular nodes

Stage 4. The presence of metastases at any distant site.

It must be stressed that this staging system is based entirely on clinical investigations and cannot take into account the presence of occult disease elsewhere which may be present and eventually become manifest as recurrent metastatic disease.

Treatment

Operable disease (Stages 1 and 2). Stages 1 and 2 breast cancer as defined above are technically completely removable by operation. These stages are therefore regarded as operable and the disease is *potentially* curable by surgery alone.

The classical operation for the treatment of operable breast cancer is the radical mastectomy described by Halsted. In this operation, the whole breast, overlying skin, pectorales major and minor muscles and the total axillary contents are removed in continuity. This operation leads to considerable deformity and sometimes permanent lymphoedema of the arm. More recently less radical procedures have been studied. The simple mastectomy (total mastectomy) involves removal of the breast and overlying skin whilst in the modified radical mastectomy the breast and axillary contents are removed leaving the pectoralis major muscle. More radical operations have also been done in which the Halsted operation has been supplemented by dissection of the internal mammary lymph nodes (super radical mastectomy). Post-operative radiotherapy to the regional lymph nodes has also been used as an adjunct to these procedures. Recently attempts have been made at conserving as much normal breast tissue as possible by performing a wide excision of the primary tumour (extended tylectomy), the remaining breast tissue being irradiated subsequently to prevent local recurrence.

In terms of patient survival, any of the above procedures gives similar results in Stage 1 disease, but with regard to local recurrence, the more radical procedures give better results. In Stage 2 disease, better survival possibly follows the more radical procedures.

The prognosis after the surgical treatment of operable breast cancer is related to the degree of axillary node involvement. In Stage 1 disease where there is no axillary involvement the recurrence rate at 5 years is about 20 per cent and the survival at this time is 76 per cent. If, however, axillary nodes are involved (Stage 2) then the recurrence rate at 5 years is as high as 66 per cent and the survival falls to 50 per cent, and if four or more nodes in the axilla are found to be involved the prognosis is much worse, there being a recurrence rate of 80 per cent at 5 years and a survival of only 30 per cent at this time.

The reason for the poor results of surgery in Stage 2 breast cancer is that in this situation, pre-clinical metastases are already present at the time of operation. Surgery is therefore unable to cure the disease and the occult metastases ultimately grow and become manifest. It is in the preclinical state that metastases are more likely to be responsive to chemotherapy by virtue of the more favourable kinetic situation as discussed in Chapter 5. The use of adjuvant chemotherapy after operation in Stage 2 breast cancer is being extensively investigated and recent evidence suggests that this may result in a decrease in the early recurrence rate of Stage 2 disease in premenopausal patients. In order to achieve these results chemotherapy may have to be prolonged and continued perhaps for one or two years after operation. Rational selection of patients for adjuvant chemotherapy needs an accurate assessment of the degree of involvement of the axillary nodes. For this reason, whatever is the primary operation, a complete axillary dissection is considered necessary until such time as better methods of predicting risk of recurrence become available. It is not yet known what effect adjuvant chemotherapy has on survival.

Paget's disease of the nipple is treated by mastectomy as discussed above for operable breast cancer provided features of Stage 3 or 4 disease are not present, in which case the treatments discussed below would be applicable.

Locally recurrent disease. After Stage 1 or 2 breast cancer has been treated, disease may recur locally. This is more likely after the less radical treatment procedures. Discrete skin nodules in, or adjacent to, the mastectomy scar are usually readily excised surgically or, if this is not possible, they can be irradiated. If the recurrence occurs in the remaining breast tissue after wide excision of a primary breast cancer, it is then usual to proceed to a total mastectomy. Axillary node recurrence is common after wide excision or simple mastectomy. These are treated either by an axillary clearance operation or radiotherapy. If locally recurrent disease is so extensive that it cannot be treated by either surgery or radiotherapy, then systemic methods of treatment discussed below for Stage 4 breast cancer become necessary.

Stage 3 disease. Primary inoperable locally advanced breast cancer (Stage 3) is treated conventionally by radiotherapy. In most cases this achieves an initial regression of the primary tumour and involved lymph nodes, but the long-term results of treatment are poor. Frequently, the local disease relapses and, in well over half of patients, distant metastases ultimately become evident. The 5-year survival in Stage 3 is less than 20 per cent.

Because local recurrence after radiotherapy is so common and cannot usually be treated by further radiotherapy, palliative mastectomy after primary radiotherapy is often performed. This reduces considerably the incidence of distressing recurrent local lesions.

In view of the high incidence of subsequent distant metastases, studies of chemotherapy in the planned initial treatment of Stage 3 breast cancer are being undertaken. It is too early to know whether this approach will improve the prognosis in Stage 3 disease.

Distant metastatic disease (Stage 4). A plan for the systemic treatment of metastatic breast cancer is shown in Fig. 8.1. Single discrete lesions are often treatable by local means but disseminated disease needs systemic therapy. Distant, but localised skin metastases may be treated by surgical excision or radiotherapy. Occasionally the only manifestation of distant disease is a pleural effusion and it may be appropriate just to treat this locally (Chapter 20). The skeleton is the most common site of distant metastases and radiotherapy is especially useful in treating localised lesions. In particular, if metastases in the spine are detected early and treated by radiotherapy they may be prevented from progressing to collapse and spinal cord compression. Radiotherapy is valuable in treating painful bony lesions by usually conferring considerable symptomatic relief. Pathological fractures of bones may occur. A Küntscher nail to strengthen a fractured

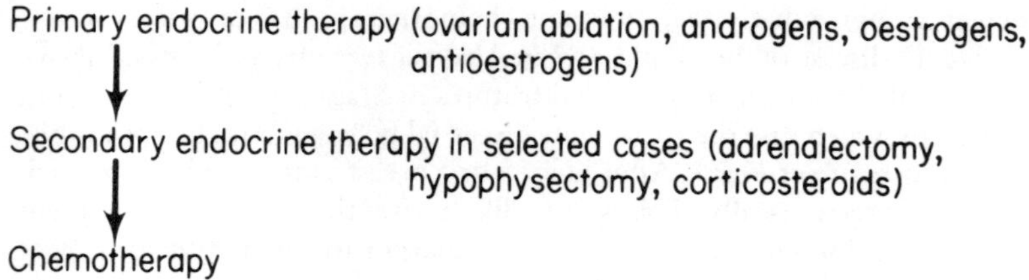

FIG. 8.1   Conventional sequential use of systemic treatments in the management of metastatic breast cancer.

femur or the replacement of the femoral head by a prosthesis may allow a patient with advanced breast cancer subsequently to enjoy considerable mobility. It is occasionally expedient to pin a long bone prophylactically if cortical erosion is marked and a pathological fracture likely to occur.

Primary endocrine therapy. Endocrine therapy is the most commonly used initial treatment for widespread breast cancer. Treatments include ovarian ablation and the administration of androgens, oestrogens or antioestrogens. In pre-menopausal women, tumour growth may be stimulated by circulating ovarian hormones and in this group of patients ovarian ablation is usually preferred. In post-menopausal women oophorectomy is of no benefit but androgens can be beneficial in the early post-menopausal period; thereafter oestrogens or antioestrogens are the preferred treatment (see below).

Ovarian ablation   This can readily be done by bilateral salpingo-oophorectomy (removal of the mesosalpinx as well as the ovaries is important as it may be the site of ectopic ovarian tissue). It is a relatively minor surgical procedure and the operation also provides an opportunity to note whether the abdominal viscera or peritoneum are involved in the disease. Ablation of ovarian function by a short course of pelvic irradiation is a suitable alternative procedure. This produces ultimately the same effect as surgical oophorectomy but takes some weeks to result in a complete cessation of ovarian hormone production. About 25 per cent of premenopausal patients undergoing ovarian ablation have some objective improvement during which soft tissue and visceral lesions regress and lytic bone deposits may recalcify. The average duration of remissions is about one year but occasionally some patients may have rather longer remissions.

Androgens   Androgens sometimes have a suppressive effect on breast-cancer growth. They are most useful in the early post-menopausal period (6 months to 5 years after the last menstrual period) but give a response rate of only about 15–20 per cent. Androgens have unwanted effects which are related to their properties as male hormones. Virilisation, associated with the development of a deeper voice and facial hair, usually occurs. but this is less of a problem with modern anabolic steroids. The commonly used androgens are nandrolone phenylpropionate (Durabolin) 25 mg weekly and fluoxymesterone (Ultandren) 20–30 mg daily. Very occasionally androgens may stimulate progression of tumour growth or hypercalcaemia may occur, in which events they must be stopped immediately.

Oestrogens   Although oestrogens may encourage the growth of breast cancer in pre-menopausal patients, in those who are more than five years post-menopausal, high doses of these hormones can confer considerable therapeutic effect. About 35 per cent of women achieve some benefit and some have very long remissions although relapse usually occurs within about two years. Older women are particularly likely to have good remission during which they may be entirely free of disease. The most commonly used oestrogen is stilboestrol 15–50 mg daily. Its administration can be associated with side-effects, including anorexia, nausea and vomiting, particularly at the beginning of therapy. These symptoms are not usually a problem and become less severe with time, but, if they are intolerable, treatment should be changed to ethinyloestradiol 0.5–1 mg daily. Fluid retention may develop and, in patients with ischaemic heart disease, cardiac failure may occur. Oestrogens may cause vaginal discharges and urinary urgency or incontinence. Rarely, oestrogens may induce the tumour to progress and hypercalcaemia may also occur. Because of their relative freedom from side-effects it is probable that anti-oestrogens will replace oestrogen therapy in the future (see below).

When patients who have had a satisfactory response to oestrogens relapse, then the discontinuation of oestrogen therapy may be associated with a further remission. This 'oestrogen withdrawal effect' may result in a patient remaining in remission for a considerable time without any treatment. A withdrawal effect is occasionally seen after other additive hormone treatments.

Anti-oestrogens   Tamoxifen, nafoxidine and clomiphene are agents which compete with oestrogens for their receptor proteins in the cytoplasm of cells and are therefore called anti-oestrogens. In the treatment of breast cancer they have been found to be therapeutically effective leading to regressions in about 30 per cent of post-menopausal patients with disseminated disease. In contrast to androgens and oestrogens they are almost free from toxic side-effects. Because of this and their equal efficacy, anti-oestrogens are now gradually replacing the other hormones as primary endocrine therapy.

Secondary endocrine therapy. Patients who have failed to respond to primary endocrine treatment or have responded and relapsed subsequently may then be considered for other endocrine ablation procedures. These are adrenalectomy and hypophysectomy. Hypophysectomy gives a higher response rate and a longer period of remission, but the choice of procedure is usually determined by the facilities available locally.

The objective response rate to secondary endocrine treatment is only 20–30 per cent and, therefore, in unselected cases will be ineffective in the majority of patients. However, by biochemical analysis of urinary steroids and expression of quantities of urinary corticosteroid and andro-gen metabolites in terms of an arithmetic ratio (urinary discriminant) it has been possible to predict which patients are most likely to benefit. Also, patients who have previously responded well to oophorectomy or who are at least six years post-menopausal and had a period free of disease after mastectomy of at least two years, are most likely to respond favour-ably to ablative procedures. In these groups the successful response rates are as high as 40 per cent and the average remission time is three years; much longer responses are occasionally obtained.

Adrenalectomy   Adrenalectomy is an operation readily performed in general surgical units and special facilities are not required. After this operation replacement therapy with glucocorticoids and often a mineralo-corticoid is needed. Normal physiological requirements for these hor-mones are satisfied by prescribing cortisone acetate 25 mg in the morning and $12\frac{1}{2}$ mg at night and 9–alpha fluorohydrocortisone up to 0.1 mg daily. After adrenalectomy, patients are liable to develop Addisonian crises in stressful situations, particularly after accidents and during anaesthetics or intercurrent illnesses. In these circumstances it is important that the corti-sone dose be increased promptly or hydrocortisone given parenterally if necessary.

Hypophysectomy   Removal of the pituitary gland (hypophysectomy) can be done in several ways. One approach is by a craniotomy (trans-frontal hypophysectomy) when the stalk joining the pituitary to the hypo-thalamus is cut and the gland removed from its fossa. Another operation avoids a craniotomy by approaching the gland through the anterior part of the fossa through the sphenoid bone (transphenoidal hypophysectomy). An alternative way of destroying pituitary function without removing the gland is irradiation by implanting radioactive yttrium into the sella turcica.

To maintain normal physiological function after hypophysectomy, certain hormones have to be replaced. Corticosteroids have to be given immediately in the same doses that are used after adrenalectomy, but re-placement of a mineralocorticoid is not needed. After complete hypophys-ectomy, patients ultimately become hypothyroid and replacement of thyroid hormone is then essential. The posterior pituitary secretes anti-diuretic hormone and, after removal of the gland, patients usually develop diabetes insipidus. This is treated by administering synthetic vasopressin as a nasal spray or desiccated animal posterior pituitary in the form of a snuff, the active agent being absorbed from the nasal mucosa. Occasion-ally it is necessary to give tablets of chlorothiazide or chlorpropamide if thirst and polyuria are not controlled adequately. Such treatment becomes less necessary with time and can often be discontinued eventually.

Apart from complications arising from the removal of important physiological hormones, hypophysectomy may be associated with other serious complications. After the transfrontal operation there is a liability to epileptiform fits (as there is after any craniotomy) and patients are routinely given phenobarbitone post-operatively. This is not a problem after transphenoidal hypophysectomy but leakage of cerebrospinal fluid through the nose can occur (cerebrospinal rhinorrhoea) resulting in meningitis. There is a risk of visual impairment after either operation.

Corticosteroids   Corticosteroids can be of some use in controlling disseminated breast cancer giving a 20 per cent response rate. It is probable that this is partly due to a suppressive effect on adrenal cortical function, although there may be some direct anti-tumour action as well. These agents can be used as an alternative to hypophysectomy or adrenalectomy and are particularly useful in patients over 65 years of age or those who are too ill for the major ablative procedures. The usual dose of prednisolone is 5 mg *t.d.s.* This is a moderate dose and is not usually associated with the well-known side-effects of corticosteroids. However, should these be troublesome the dosage can be reduced.

Other hormonal therapies. Progestational agents such as norethisterone acetate and medroxyprogesterone are sometimes able to suppress temporarily the growth of breast cancer and response rates of between 20 and 30 per cent have been reported. The mechanism of action of progestogens in breast cancer, although not known, may be due to a suppression of gonadotrophin secretion or a direct effect on the tumour. Norethisterone acetate is given in a dose of 10–20 mg *t.d.s.* which is not usually associated with serious untoward side-effects. Mild fluid retention with weight gain and vaginal bleeding may occur. Rarely cholestatic jaundice occurs which resolves on stopping the drug. Occasionally stimulation, rather than suppression, of tumour growth is induced.

Other, less successful, forms of endocrine therapy have been used in the treatment of advanced breast cancer. These include aminoglutethimide (which suppresses the synthesis of adrenal hormones by blocking the conversion of cholesterol to pregnenolone) and bromocryptine (which suppresses prolactin secretion, the relevance of which to human breast cancer is not known).

Chemotherapy. Unlike other common carcinomas, breast cancer is responsive to a variety of cytotoxic drugs which have been traditionally reserved until endocrine therapy has failed. Used as single agents, the drugs cyclophosphamide, methotrexate and fluorouracil can produce responses in 30–40 per cent of women with advanced breast cancer, while others, notably the vinca alkaloids, cause responses in about 20 per cent of patients. These drugs used in combination are more effective in producing remissions, which are of longer duration, than when the agents are used singly with response rates of over 50 per cent being reported. Recently doxorubicin (Adriamycin) has been introduced into clinical use, and this now appears to be the most effective drug in breast cancer and used alone induces remissions in 45 per cent or more of patients. This drug is probably even more effective in combination with other agents. Current effective combinations include: (a) cyclophosphamide + methotrexate + 5-fluorouracil ± vinca alkaloids ± prednisone; (b) Adriamycin + vincristine; and (c) Adriamycin + cyclophosphamide ± 5-fluorouracil. An example of one of these regimens is shown in Fig. 8.2.

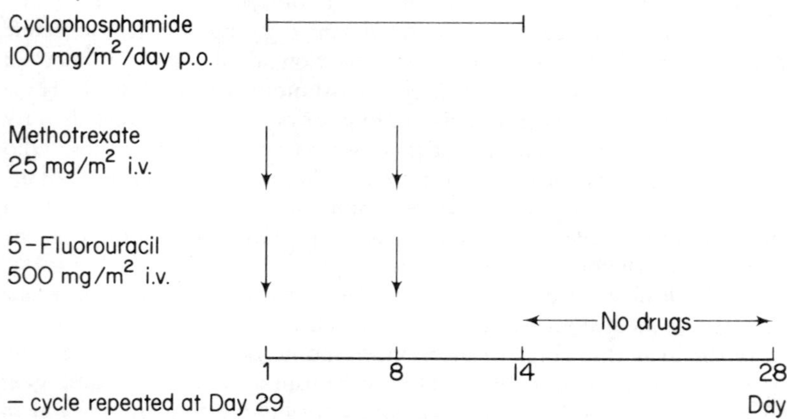

FIG. 8.2 The 'CMF' regimen for advanced breast cancer. The doses given are approximate, optimal doses are determined by age and blood counts.

Chemotherapy in breast cancer has now made considerable advances and with modern combinations response rates over 60 per cent are achieved with remissions lasting over a year. For this reason chemotherapy is now being used at an earlier stage in many centres, particularly in preference to the major ablation procedures of hypophysectomy and adrenalectomy.

Prediction of response to therapy. In advanced breast cancer, successes from any one treatment are limited to a minority of cases. Many patients receive treatment from which they derive no benefit, but which nevertheless was given because of the possibility of a response. For this reason attempts are being made to develop tests to predict whether or not a patient will respond to treatment. Factors indicating a favourable response to hypophysectomy have already been mentioned. A promising recent development is a test to detect whether cells in a tumour contain oestrogen-binding proteins (oestrogen receptors). When oestrogen receptors are absent it is very improbable that a patient will respond to hormone therapy and she can be saved unnecessary treatment, but when these receptors are detected then there is an approximately 50 per cent chance of responding to endocrine therapy. This is rather better than the response rates for endocrine treatments mentioned above when given without knowledge of tumour receptor contents.

These analyses, which depend on the availability of fresh tumour tissue, are not yet widely available and their precise role in selecting systemic therapy for advanced disease remains to be determined. Recent evidence suggests that concomitant measurement of progesterone receptors is likely to improve the power of prediction of these tests.

There is a direct relationship between receptor positivity and the differentiation of the tumour and it has been suggested that the more anaplastic, proliferative oestrogen-receptor-negative tumours will be somewhat more sensitive to cytotoxic chemotherapy than tumours positive for these receptors. It is thus likely that these tests will have an important role in the future in selecting the most appropriate systemic treatment for patients with disseminated breast cancer.

Screening for breast cancer

It is probable that the earlier breast cancer can be detected then the more likely it is to be curable by treatment. This has led to the establishment of screening programmes in which asymptomatic women can be examined in order to detect the presence of relatively early disease. The methods employed include clinical examination, breast radiography (mammography and xeroradiography) and thermography. The problems of screening large asymptomatic populations are formidable. The economic costs are large and any benefits must be weighed against such factors as irradiation risks from mammography (low with modern techniques), unnecessary biopsies, which will inevitably occur, and the generation of anxiety. Furthermore, it is essential that treatment of lesions detected on screening should lead to a real increase in cure rate, not just an apparent increase in survival as a result of earlier diagnosis. Recent evidence suggests that screening women over the age of 50 years can partly achieve this. It is probable that for screening to be effective and economically feasible it will have to be restricted to women identified as having a high risk of developing the disease.

CHAPTER NINE

BLOOD AND BONE MARROW

The various malignancies affecting blood and bone marrow are, individually, uncommon, but together form a large group of diseases. They differ widely from each other with regard both to clinical features and management. Their aetiology is generally unknown, but there is an increased incidence of acute leukaemia after previous exposure to irradiation (e.g. radiotherapy for ankylosing spondylitis, atomic bomb explosions) and with certain chromosomal disorders, particularly Down's syndrome (mongolism).

LEUKAEMIAS

The term leukaemia refers specifically to an excess of white blood cells in the blood, but the term is more loosely used to apply to an abnormal increase in any of the blood cells (e.g. erythroleukaemia, megakaryocytic leukaemia). This section will deal with malignant proliferative disorders affecting the white blood cells.

Acute lymphoblastic leukaemia

This is the most common malignant disease of childhood. Its highest incidence is at about 5 years of age and it is rare after 15 years. The disease is characterised by an excessive proliferation of immature lymphocytes (lymphoblasts) in the bone marrow and peripheral blood. In 70–80 per cent of cases, these lymphoblasts ('null-cells') lack immunological features of T or B cells, but most of the remaining cases show T-cell markers suggesting a thymic origin. These T-cell leukaemias are associated with mediastinal tumours (Sternberg's sarcoma) and have a particularly poor prognosis.

Clinical features

Symptoms include malaise, weight loss, fever and anorexia, and haemorrhagic manifestations (e.g. bleeding gums) may occur. Bone and joint pains are common. Physical examination usually shows some enlargement of lymph nodes and spleen with pallor and bruising. There may be signs of infection—for example in the throat skin, or respiratory tract.

Meningeal infiltration (meningeal leukaemia) which is quite common, leads to symptoms and signs of raised intracranial pressure (headache, vomiting and papilloedema). Examination of the cerebro-spinal fluid shows an increased protein content, and the presence of leukaemic cells. Occasionally spinal-cord compression may occur producing a paraplegia.

Investigations

The peripheral blood count shows a leukocytosis up to 20–$30 \times 10^9/l$ due to an excess of lymphoblasts. Marrow suppression usually produces anaemia and thrombocytopenia. The diagnosis is confirmed by marrow examination. A blood picture resembling that of acute lymphoblastic leukaemia (leukaemoid reaction) is sometimes found in certain benign conditions (e.g. infectious mononucleosis, pertussis, and miliary tuberculosis) although the reason for this is not known.

Treatment

Major advances have been made in the management of this condition in the last decade. It was in this disease that combination chemotherapy was pioneered and its effectiveness established. The aim of treatment is first to induce a complete remission, when all detectable disease in the blood and bone marrow disappears, and then to maintain this remission with further treatment. Complete remission in this disease is attainable in over 90 per cent of patients using a combination of vincristine and prednisone. This remission is then best maintained with either methotrexate or 6-mercaptopurine. Although systemic chemotherapy may maintain remission in the blood and bone marrow, relapse with meningeal disease occurs in many patients unless prophylactic treatment to the central nervous system is given after haematological remission has been achieved. The preferred method is cranial irradiation together with intrathecal methotrexate but, alternatively, the spinal meninges too may be irradiated.

Acute lymphoblastic leukaemia in adults is treated similarly but the results are less satisfactory. This disease in adults may be a facet of diffuse poorly differentiated lymphocytic lymphoma (see Chapter 10).

More than half of the children with this once invariably fatal disease now have disease-free periods after treatment of five years or more, and can probably be considered cured. Poor prognosis is associated with mediastinal, meningeal and testicular involvement and with high initial lymphoblast counts, particularly if the cells exhibit markers indicating a thymic origin.

Acute myeloblastic leukaemia

Unlike lymphoblastic leukaemia, this disease is not clearly age-related, although it is predominantly a disease of adults. Acute myeloblastic leukaemia is characterised by the replacement of the bone marrow with immature cells of myeloid series. This disorder is occasionally associated with other haematological disturbances, such as sideroblastic anaemia, aplastic anaemia and paroxysmal nocturnal haemoglobinuria. The terminal stage of myelofibrosis sometimes resembles acute myeloblastic leukaemia. Several sporadic case reports have suggested that prolonged treatment with cytotoxic drugs, for example in the treatment of Hodgkin's disease, may predispose to the development of this leukaemia.

Clinical features

The clinical features are non-specific and include general malaise, fever and weight loss. Haemorrhagic manifestations such as bleeding gums, bruising and fundal haemorrhages are seen on physical examination. The spleen is often palpable, but lymph-node enlargement is rare.

Investigations

Peripheral blood count shows anaemia, thrombocytopenia and, despite the elevation of white-cell count due to the presence of immature myeloblasts, there is a neutropenia. Bone-marrow examination shows a marked infiltration of the marrow by abnormal myeloblasts and the normal blood-cell precursors are greatly reduced. Occasionally myeloblasts are found only in the marrow, but not in the peripheral blood (aleukaemic leukaemia). Sometimes the blood picture in other conditions (e.g. certain infections) may also resemble acute myeloblastic leukaemia because of circulating immature granulocytes. Certain enzyme stains (e.g. for peroxide and alkaline phosphatase) may assist in recognition of the cellular origin of the disease. Due to a high rate of nucleic acid turn-over hyperuricaemia is common.

Depending on the morphological appearance of the abnormal myeloblasts, other variants of acute myeloblastic leukaemia are described. These include acute promyelocytic, myelomonocytic and monocytic leukaemias. When the myeloblastic proliferation is accompanied by a predominance of abnormal cells of the erythroid series, the term erythroleukaemia (Di Guglielmo's disease) is applied.

Treatment

Treatment aims at eradicating the abnormal myeloblasts and allowing the normal marrow to proliferate. This is achieved temporarily in about 50 per cent of cases using a combination of daunorubicin and cytosine arabinoside. This disease is less sensitive to other cytotoxic agents, but may respond to combinations of drugs in which the following may be used: 6-mercaptopurine, methotrexate, prednisone, vincristine, L-asparaginase, cyclophosphamide, 6-thioguanine. Remission induction is accompanied by high nucleic acid destruction and elevation of blood urate so that allopurinol should be given prophylactically during treatment to avoid the occurrence of acute gout and nephropathy. Until cytotoxic therapy was available the survival in this disease after diagnosis was about 2 months, but the remissions now obtained with chemotherapy have extended the survival of some pateients for over a year.

Immunotherapy with BCG and irradiated allogeneic leukaemic cells may prolong remission but this form of treatment is controversial and should only be given in controlled clinical trials.

Supportive therapy is particularly important in acute myeloblastic leukaemia in the form of antibiotic therapy for the frequent infections which occur and transfusions to correct anaemia and thrombocytopenia. Reverse barrier nursing may be of value in controlling infections and in specialised centres, leukocyte transfusions can be given.

Chronic lymphocytic leukaemia (chronic lymphatic leukaemia)

This is predominantly a disease of middle and old age. Unlike the other leukaemias, where there is no marked sex difference, this disease is twice as common in males as in females. Chronic lymphocytic leukaemia is characterised by the abnormal proliferation and prolonged survival of mature small lymphocytes which circulate in the blood and aggregate in lymph nodes and the spleen.

Clinical features and investigations

The onset of this disease is insidious. The uncomplicated disease is not usually associated with constitutional disturbance and may be found by chance on routine blood examination. Superficial lymph-node enlargement usually brings the disease to notice, and this is confirmed on physical examination which shows marked lymphadenopathy in all superficial node areas together with hepatosplenomegaly. Complications arise when infiltration of the marrow by small lymphocytes becomes so excessive as to suppress blood formation, or if tumour masses cause pressure symptoms.

Haemolytic anaemia is common and may be rapid in onset. Alternatively, it may develop so slowly that extremely low haemoglobin levels (e.g. below 5 g/100 ml) are reached before the condition is recognised. Patients are prone to infections (Chapter 22). The peripheral blood shows a marked increase in small lymphocytes, counts in excess of $30 \times 10^9/l$ being common. Occasionally, the lymphocytosis may be extreme and white blood cell counts of $1 \times 10^{12}/l$ or more are not unknown. Marrow examination and lymph node biopsy show infiltration by small lymphocytes.

Treatment

This disease sometimes appears to be a facet of diffuse, well-differentiated lymphocytic lymphoma (Chapter 10), and treatment may not be required unless complications appear. These include suppression of haematopoiesis, haemolytic anaemia (usually Coombs positive) and pressure from lymph-node masses. A rising lymphocyte count is also an indication for treatment when it exceeds $100 \times 10^9/l$, because at this level complications are probable. The disease is then usually readily controlled by chlorambucil and prednisolone, guided by periodical blood counts. Recent studies of whole-body irradiation have suggested that this treatment produces worthwhile remissions in this disease. Haemolytic anaemia is treated by the administration of corticosteroids. Radiotherapy is useful for the treatment of lymph-node masses and occasionally of splenomegaly. Chronic lymphocytic leukaemia is often a protracted condition which can be controlled by simple therapy, the patient often leading a relatively normal life for several years.

Chronic myeloid leukaemia (chronic granulocytic leukaemia)

This disease is rare before the age of 20 and the incidence increases with age. Chronic myeloid leukaemia is a proliferative disorder of marrow stem cells affecting principally the granulocytes. A constant chromosomal abnormality occurs in which there is a deletion in the long arm of chromosome 21 called the Philadelphia chromosome. This chromosomal abnormality is seen in dividing cells of the erythroid and megakaryocytic, as well as the granulocytic, series. Initially, chronic myeloid leukaemia is an indolent disease and the malignant cells are well-differentiated. The disease, however, always ends in an acute terminal phase in which immature blast cells predominate (blast-cell transformation; blast-cell crisis).

Clinical features

This disease has an insidious onset or may sometimes be discovered on routine examination. General malaise and abdominal discomfort due to splenomegaly are the principal symptoms. Examination shows marked splenic enlargement in most patients, but lymph node or hepatic enlargement is unusual. There may be bleeding tendencies due to poor platelet function. In the terminal blast-cell phase the patient becomes ill with fever, bone pain and increasing spleen size. Localised tumour masses, due to the aggregation of neoplastic cells (chloromas), may be seen. Death follows within a few weeks of the appearance of the blast-cell crisis.

Investigations

The peripheral blood shows a leukocytosis due to a marked increase in well-differentiated granulocytes. The white-cell count is usually in excess of $30 \times 10^9/l$ and may reach $300 \times 10^9/l$ or more. Anaemia is frequent but platelets are either normal or in excess and there may be an increase in circulating immature white cells, nucleated red cells, eosinophils or basophils. Occasionally, basophils or eosinophils are the predominant cell. Because of the high turn-over of nucleic acids, the blood urate is usually elevated.

Treatment

The aim of treatment in chronic myeloid leukaemia is to suppress haematopoiesis sufficiently for the patient to become asymptomatic. This is usually readily achieved by administering busulphan orally. Treatment may be associated with an increase in hyperuricaemia and allopurinol should be administered concommitantly. This simple therapy enables most patients to enjoy good health for some years, but blast-cell transformation invariably occurs. Attempts to treat this as acute myeloblastic leukaemia are generally unsuccessful. However, recent evidence has shown a relationship between blast-cell crisis and lymphoblastic leukaemia, suggesting that more appropriate treatment may be to employ vincristine and prednisone. Splenectomy in the primary management of chronic myeloid leukaemia in order to delay blast transformation has been investigated and is probably of minimal value.

POLYCYTHAEMIA RUBRA VERA

Polycythaemia rubra vera is a myeloproliferative disorder in which there is an increased production of all the formed elements of the blood. The clinical disturbance, however, is largely due to an excess of red blood cells. The majority of cases occur between the ages of 40 and 70 years.

Clinical features

The clinical features are due to the increased blood volume and viscosity causing engorgement of organs and slowing of the circulation. Commonly there is headache, dizziness, tinnitus and poor concentration, while sometimes cerebral infarction occurs. Cardiorespiratory symptoms are frequent, half the patients having raised blood pressure and many suffering from angina, sometimes myocardial infarction, or dyspnoea due to congestive cardiac failure. Thrombocythaemia contributes to arterial and venous (superficial or deep) thrombosis. Despite increased platelet counts, haemorrhagic manifestations are seen particularly as epistaxes, gastrointestinal bleeding or bruising. Itching is a common symptom although its cause is unknown. Peptic ulceration is a frequent association, as are visual disturbances, bone pain and general malaise. Patients have a plethoric or cyanotic appearance; superficial telangiectases may be seen, splenomegaly is usual and ophthalmoscopic examination shows retinal vessel engorgement. Gout is a common complication due to associated hyperuricaemia. Common causes of death in polycythaemia are the various complications of haemorrhage or thrombosis and the disease may terminate as myelofibrosis or acute myeloblastic leukaemia.

Investigations

The red blood cell count is high ($8\text{--}9 \times 10^{12}/l$ or greater), the haemoglobin is commonly $18\text{--}24$ g/dl and the packed cell volume 60–70 per cent, usually with a small increase in reticulocytes. A useful investigation is estimation of red cell mass by an isotopic technique. There is elevation of the white blood count ($12\text{--}20 \times 10^{9}/l$ per mm^3) and the leukocyte alkaline phosphatase is raised, which distinguishes polycythaemia rubra vera from secondary polycythaemia (see below). The platelet count is characteristically in the range $500–1000 \times 10^9/l$ but may be considerably higher. The erythrocyte sedimentation rate is low. There is usually some elevation of serum bilirubin and blood uric acid is high. Bone-marrow examination shows a generalised hyperplasia. Marrow scintiscan reveals intra- and extra- medullary extension of normal areas of erythropoiesis.

Differential diagnosis

Polycythaemia rubra vera should be distinguished from secondary polycythaemia, which may occur as an excessive response to hypoxaemia (as in Fallot's tetralogy or, sometimes, chronic obstructive lung disease) or to the excessive production of erythropoietin in renal carcinoma, primary liver cancer, cerebellar haemangioblastoma and uterine myomata. In secondary polycythaemia the leukocyte alkaline phosphatase is normal.

Treatment

Rapid relief of symptoms is achieved most efficiently and maintained by regular venesection of 500 ml daily until the haematocrit is reduced to 50 per cent. The most well-established treatment, to correct excessive proliferation of bone marrow cells, is the administration of radioactive phosphorus (^{32}P) which is taken up into the skeleton as phosphate. ^{32}P is a beta emitter and the bone marrow is selectively irradiated. This effectively inhibits bone marrow activity and leads to a resolution of the clinical manifestations. There are no immediate toxic effects from this treatment, but some evidence suggests that the incidence of leukaemia is greater after ^{32}P therapy. It is possible, however, that the prolonged survival, which appears to be achieved by this therapy, increases the chance of terminal leukaemia developing, rather than it being caused by the radioactive isotope. If symptoms, or elevation of the packed cell volume recur, then ^{32}P therapy can be repeated. Alkylating agents are useful in the treatment of this condition and achieve similar results to radioactive phosphorus. The true place of these therapies in polycythaemia rubra vera has not yet been established finally and a controlled trial comparing venesection, radioactive phosphorus and bulsulphan is in progress.

MYELOFIBROSIS

This is a disorder in which the bone marrow becomes replaced by fibrous tissue or sometimes even bone. This can happen in association with a variety of pre-existing conditions (e.g. osseous metastases, certain infections, chemical poisons) in which case it is called secondary myelofibrosis, or it may occur as a primary condition.

The principal features are a leukoerythroblastic anaemia and characteristic 'tear drop' poikilocytes in the peripheral blood with evidence of extra-medullary erythropoiesis. The spleen is usually large. Marrow aspiration usually fails and trephine biopsy reveals the increased fibrosis.

Although the disease in its typical form usually has a long course over years, there is a variety referred to as malignant myelofibrosis in which there is rapid deterioration with severe anaemia, neutropenia and thrombocytopenia.

Treatment consists of blood transfusion and supportive measures together with therapy for the underlying disease. In the primary form, folic acid and anabolic steroids may produce a rise in haemoglobin level. Sometimes corticosteroid therapy is useful.

PLASMA-CELL TUMOURS

Excessive plasma-cell formation leads to a variety of clinical conditions. Plasma cells, which are derived from the ultimate differentiation of B-lymphocytes, are immunoglobulin-producing cells and tumours arising from them are characterised by the presence of high levels of circulating immunoglobulins. These conditions are sometimes referred to as paraproteinaemias. Individual plasma-cell tumours are derived from single clones of cells (monoclonal origin) and the immunoglobulin produced in excess is of a single molecular type (the M-protein) and identified as a discrete band on plasma electrophoresis.

In myelomatosis the malignant plasma cells are usually confined to the bone marrow. The effects of the disease are seen mainly in the blood and skeleton, and also as a result of the M-protein. Rarely, localised extra-medullary plasma-cell tumours occur. Other paraproteinaemias such as Waldenströms macroglobulinaemia are clinically similar to the malignant lymphomas and these are discussed in Chapter 10.

Myelomatosis (multiple myeloma)

This is the most common plasma-cell tumour and is seen in middle and late life.

Clinical features

Weakness, loss of weight, bone pain and increased susceptibility to infections are common. Extensive destruction of bones occurs leading to pathological fractures and vertebral collapse which in some cases may cause paraplegia. The M-protein may cause the hyperviscosity syndrome (Chapter 10). Renal failure is common and is due to several factors: deposition of paraprotein in the tubules, hypercalcaemia, hyperuricaemia or a combination of these, and may be precipitated by dehydration. Amyloidosis sometimes complicates myelomatosis.

Investigations

The peripheral blood commonly shows a normochromic normocytic anaemia, occasionally circulating plasma cells are seen (plasma cell leukaemia), and bone-marrow examination shows infiltration by plasma cells. Plasma electrophoresis shows a discrete band in the gammaglobulin fraction, confirming a monoclonal origin of the M-protein which is usually of the IgM, IgA or IgG type in increasing order of frequency; IgD and IgE myelomas are exceedingly rare. Extra-medullary plasmacytomas, which are sometimes situated in mucous membranes, are usually associated with IgA production. Immunoglobulin light chains are found in the plasma and these are filtered at the glomeruli, giving rise to Bence-Jones' proteinuria. Other biochemical investigations frequently show raised blood urea and creatinine, an apparent hyponatraemia (due to plasma volume increase as a result of the hyperproteinaemia), elevated alkaline phosphatase (in reaction to bone destruction), hypercalcaemia and hyperuricaemia.

Radiologically, there are widespread lytic areas throughout the skeleton which have frequently a clear-cut punched-out appearance, particularly in the skull and ribs. The spine shows generalised osteoporosis with vertebral collapse. In those patients with renal failure, intravenous urography, if required, should be done with great caution to avoid dehydration.

Treatment

General supportive measures are important in the treatment of myelomatosis. Adequate hydration should be ensured because of the risk of patients developing renal failure. Hypercalcaemia (Chapter 21) and infections (Chapter 22) require specific treatment and plasmaphoresis is occasionally required for the hyperviscosity syndrome. Radiotherapy is of particular use for relieving pain in well-localised areas of bone involvement, while orthopaedic surgical procedures are sometimes needed to treat or prevent pathological fractures. Well-fitting spinal supports are of considerable assistance to many patients.

Specific antitumour therapy involves the use of the alkylating agents and prednisolone. Currently, the best results are obtained with Melphalan and prednisolone in combination given intermittently. Between a third and a half of patients respond well to this treatment as shown by a decrease in M-protein, increases in haemoglobin and weight, reduced susceptibility to infections and improvement in renal function.

Although the majority of patients with myelomatosis are helped greatly by treatment, they eventually die from complications of the disease. The principal causes of death are infections, particularly pneumonia, cardiac and renal failure.

CHAPTER TEN

LYMPHATIC TISSUE

Tumours of lymphatic tissue include Hodgkin's disease, other malignant lymphomas (colloquially referred to as 'non-Hodgkin's lymphomas'), Waldenströms macroglobulinaemia and Burkitt's lymphoma.

HODGKIN'S DISEASE

Hodgkin's disease is distinguished from other malignant lymphomas by the possession of a characteristic malignant cell (Reed–Sternberg cell) and by its more orderly pattern of spread. This relatively uncommon malignancy is more common in males than females and occurs predominantly in young adults with a second smaller peak in middle age. The aetiology is unknown, but recent evidence has indicated that prolonged and close person-to-person associations may be important (suggesting the possibility of a transmissible causative agent), although this is controversial. There is a higher incidence of this disease within five years of an attack of infectious mononucleosis.

Pathology

The diagnosis of Hodgkin's disease depends upon the demonstration histologically of Reed–Sternberg cells in the tumour. These are multinucleate giant cells, sometimes referred to as 'owl eye' cells. Four histological categories of Hodgkin's disease are described:

1 **Lymphocyte predominant.**
Lymphocytes are the predominant cells in this type with scanty Reed–Sternberg cells. This suggest that an immunological reaction by the host may have developed against the tumour.
2 **Nodular sclerosis.**
This type of Hodgkin's disease is characterised by marked fibrosis; the lymph nodes are seen to be subdivided by fibrous bands.
3 **Mixed cellularity.**
In addition to Reed–Sternberg cells the lymphoid tissue is infiltrated by other cells including lymphocytes, histiocytes, plasma cells and eosinophils.
4 **Lymphocyte depleted.**
Few lymphocytes are present and there is a large proportion of Reed–Sternberg cells. This possibly reflects a deficient immunological reaction against the malignant cells.

Hodgkin's disease usually appears to arise in one group of lymph nodes and then spreads to an adjacent group. If untreated, further spread to more distant nodes occurs and the spleen becomes involved. Other structures, particularly the liver, are affected later in the disease. Lymphocyte-predominant and nodular-sclerosing Hodgkin's disease may remain localised to one or two groups of nodes for a long time, but in lymphocyte depleted disease spread is more rapid and wide dissemination may have occurred at the time of presentation.

Clinical features

The patient may simply complain of a painless swelling of lymph nodes. Other symptoms occur, particularly with lymphocyte-depleted disease, and during relapse after treatment. These include fever, pruritus, general malaise, night sweats and weight loss. Pain following the consumption of alcohol is an occasional complaint. Symptoms may also arise as a result of the pressure of tumour masses on other organs, for example in the mediastinum causing cough or dyspnoea.

Physical examination shows enlargement of lymph nodes in one or more superficial node areas (cervical, axillary, epitrochlear, inguinal) and liver and/or spleen enlargement may be found. Jaundice occurs with bile duct obstruction or hepatic infiltration.

Investigations

Haematological tests may disclose the presence of anaemia and the erythrocyte sedimentation rate may be raised. Biopsy of the bone marrow rarely shows infiltration by Hodgkin's disease. Serological tests for infectious mononucleosis and toxoplasmosis should be done to exclude an infective cause for the lymphadenopathy.

A chest radiograph may demonstrate enlargement of hilar and paratracheal lymph nodes and lymphography involvement of pelvic and para-aortic nodes. An intravenous urogram performed with the lymphogram sometimes shows displacement of the ureters by the tumour. Scintiscans of the liver and spleen are of value and gallium scans occasionally demonstrate disease at other sites.

Biopsy of the tumour and histological examination are essential to confirm the diagnosis of Hodgkin's disease. Laparotomy is then undertaken in many centres, the purpose of which is to remove the spleen, sample intra-abdominal lymph nodes and biopsy the liver for further histological examination. A laparotomy may seem an extensive investigative procedure, but the advantage gained in increasing the accuracy of staging outweighs the risks. It can probably be omitted, however, in patients with Stage I lymphocyte-predominant disease and those with Stage IIIB and IV (see below). The effect of investigations on staging Hodgkin's disease is listed in Fig. 10.1.

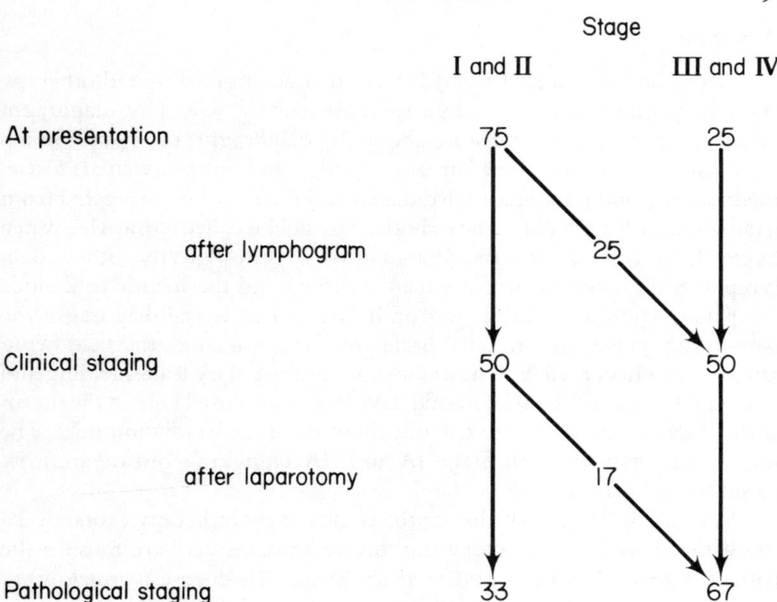

FIG. 10.1 Effect of lymphography and laparotomy on changing the apparent staging in 100 patients with Hodgkin's disease. After Aisenberg, A. C. *New Engl. J. Med.* 299, 1278, 1978.

Staging

After clinical assessment and the above investigations, Hodgkin's disease is staged according to its extent:

Stage I. Disease confined to one group of lymph nodes.

Stage II. Involvement of more than one group of lymph nodes, either above *or* below the diaphragm but not both.

Stage III. Disease confined to lymph nodes on both sides of the diaphragm, with or without splenic involvement.

Stage IV. The disease is widely disseminated, having spread beyond the lymph nodes and spleen to extra-lymphatic sites. However, for localised extralymphatic spread an alternative staging (Ann Arbor Classification) allows a lower staging to be given according to the nodal involvement qualified by the Suffix 'E', i.e. Stage I_E II_E or III_E.

The prognosis of Hodgkin's disease is adversely affected by the presence of the symptoms weight loss, night sweats and fever. This is taken into account in staging. When these symptoms are absent the stage is given the suffix A, but B if one or more are present.

Treatment

Stage I and II. Stages IA and IIA are treated entirely by radiotherapy and it is essential that all the lymph-node areas on the side of the diaphragm involved are treated. For disease above the diaphragm, the lymph nodes on both sides of the neck, in both axillae and infraclavicular fossae, mediastinum and lung hila are irradiated and the lungs are protected from irradiation by lead shields. The radiotherapy field is called a **mantle**. When Stage II disease above the diaphragm is histologically other than lymphocyte predominant it is expedient to extend the mantle to include the para-aortic nodes. In Stage I or II disease below the diaphragm the para-aortic, pelvic and inguinal node areas are irradiated, the field being known as an **inverted Y**. The kidneys are protected by lead shielding and in young females the ovaries should have been transposed behind the uterus at the staging laparotomy to exclude them from the irradiation field. The majority of patients with Stage IA and IIA Hodgkin's disease are now cured by radiotherapy alone.

Stage III. In Stage IIIA disease the results of radiotherapy ('total nodal irradiation') are less satisfactory and this treatment is very arduous for the patient. Chemotherapy is preferred for Stage IIIB disease (see below).

Stage IV. Stage IV disease is treated by chemotherapy and, in the past, single agents were used sequentially. An important advance was made when mustine, vincristine (Oncovin), procarbazine and prednisone were combined. This combination, which is widely known by the acronym MOPP, is given in four-weekly cycles (see Chapter 5, page 43) and treatment is normally continued for six courses. Further courses may prolong remission although this is not certain, but it is unlikely that survival is prolonged. Most patients with Stage IV disease achieve complete regression on this treatment and a proportion are free of disease 10 years later. Should Stage IV disease be resistant to MOPP or relapse after a response, then other drugs may be used. The non-cross-resistant combination of adriamycin, bleomycin, vinblastine and dacarbazine has given good results, and other drugs (e.g. nitrosoureas) are also of value.

The past decade has seen major advances in the management of Hodgkin's disease. This once invariably fatal condition is now one where the majority of cases are cured, the remainder obtaining considerable benefit with modern treatment. It is stressed that for this to be achieved the treatment must be adequate both with regard to dosage and duration.

NON-HODGKIN'S LYMPHOMAS

The group of diseases known collectively as non-Hodgkin's lymphomas includes a variety of conditions with differing prognoses. They differ from Hodgkin's disease in that the Reed–Sternberg cell is not present and their mode of spread is less orderly. The general clinical features are, however, similar and the same investigations are appropriate, except that laparotomy is less frequently performed.

For many years the malignant lymphomas were known by such names as giant follicular lymphoma, lymphosarcoma, and reticulum cell sarcoma. This terminology proved unsatisfactory as it did not correlate well with the natural history of these conditions, nor with their response to treatment. The malignant lymphomas have now been classified more rationally on the basis of the predominant cell type, differentiation and cellular pattern within the lymph node. This modern classification facilitates a better understanding of the prognosis and treatment of these conditions.

Based on a consideration of the two principal cell types found in lymphoid tissue, lymphocytes and histiocytes, a lymphoma may be described as being lymphocytic or histiocytic, depending on the cells involved in the malignant process. Immunological tests frequently show the malignant cells in lymphocytic lymphoma to have B-cell markers. Occasionally both lymphocytes and histiocytes are involved and the lymphoma is termed mixed. The proliferating malignant cells may be either well- or poorly-differentiated and their arrangement in the lymph nodes may be nodular or diffuse. The classification of the malignant lymphomas based on these considerations is summarised in Fig. 10.2 which also shows their relation to the older terminology.

Nodular lymphomas

Lymphomas with a nodular pattern tend to be relatively benign and, with the exception of nodular poorly-differentiated lymphomas, have better prognoses than their counterparts with diffuse histological pattern. These lymphomas were previously included in the term 'giant follicular lymphoma' (Brill–Symmers' disease).

Well-localised nodular lymphomas can be treated adequately by radiotherapy, but for widespread disease a good result is usually obtained with single alkylating agents such as chlorambucil, and it is sometimes expedient to add prednisone. This simple, non-toxic therapy usually achieves a remission which may last for many years even when treatment is stopped. However, these lymphomas occasionally recur with features of a more malignant type, and in this instance more radical treatment as for the diffuse poorly differentiated lymphomas is appropriate. Nodular poorly differentiated lymphomas are probably best treated, at the outset, by intensive combination chemotherapy.

Diffuse lymphomas

Well-differentiated lymphocytic lymphoma

Here the proliferative process involves well-differentiated small lymphocytes which fill and enlarge lymph nodes. The excess lymphocytes may also be seen in the blood, the disease then being indistinguishable from chronic lymphocytic leukaemia (p. 89).

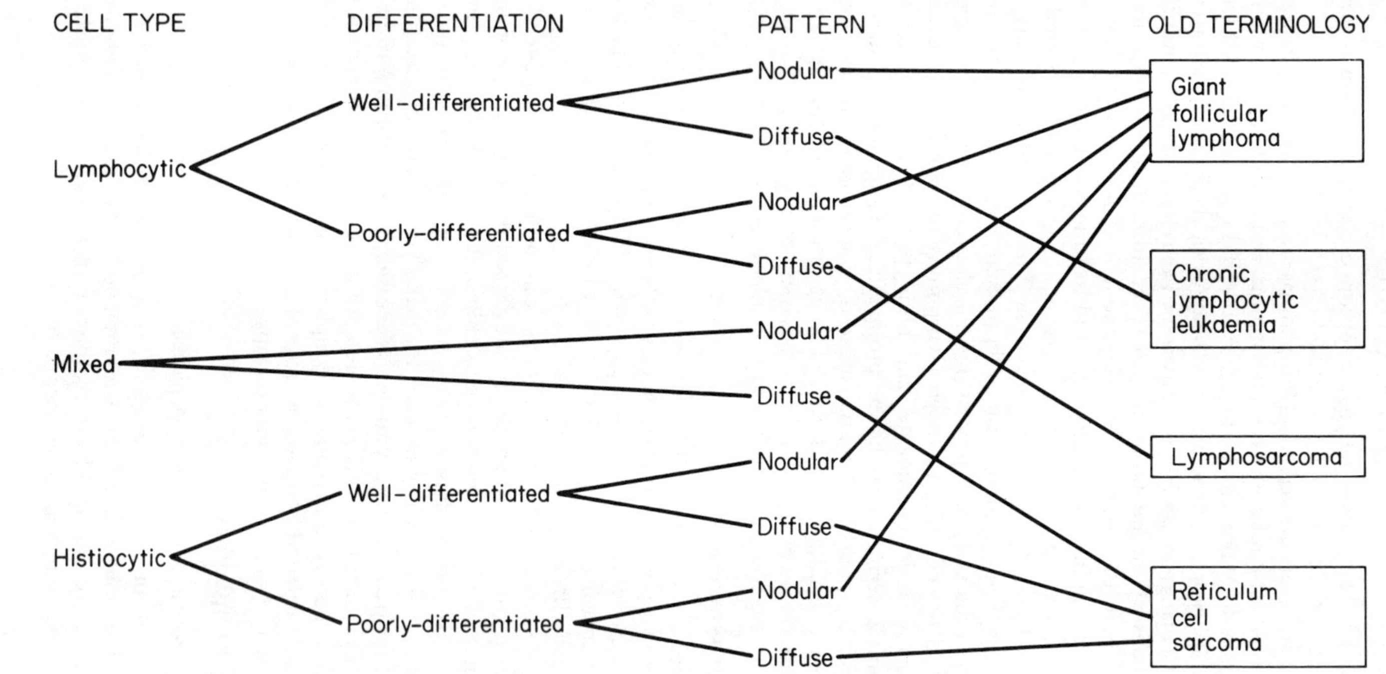

Fig. 10.2   Classification of the malignant lymphomas.

This type of lymphoma has a protracted course and a relatively good prognosis. It often does not require specific treatment unless there are complicating features which include pressure symptoms from large lymph-node masses, infections due to immunological deficiency, haemolytic anaemia or bone-marrow suppression from infiltration. The disease then usually responds to single alkylating agents such as chlorambucil or prednisone.

Waldenströms macroglobulinaemia

This is a diffuse well-differentiated lymphocytic lymphoma in which the lymphocytes involved in the proliferative disorder produce large quantities of an immunoglobulin of the IgM type (macroglobulin). In addition to a generalised lymphadenopathy and splenic enlargement there is usually marked infiltration of the bone marrow by lymphocytes and a peripheral lymphocytosis. Serum electrophoresis shows a discrete band in the gamma-globulin fraction, indicating that the abnormal proliferating lymphocytes which produce it are derived from a single clone of cells. The plasma-protein concentration may be in excess 5 g/l and this is largely responsible for the frequent occurrence of the hyperviscosity syndrome in this condition. This is characterised by general malaise, headache, nausea, dizziness and, occasionally, convulsions and coma. Haemorrhagic manifestations such as epistaxis, bleeding gums and rectal bleeding may occur. Bruising occurs easily and there is plethora and palmar erythema. The optic fundi show characteristically venous engorgement, haemorrhages, exudates and papilloedema. It is important that this condition be promptly recognised as the syndrome can be rapidly reversed by plasmaphoresis. Definitive treatment of Waldenströms macroglobulinaemia depends upon the response of the underlying conditions to systemic therapy, and/or corticosteroids. Other paraproteinaemias such as heavy-chain disease and alpha-chain disease are rare associations of lymphoproliferative disorders.

Diffuse poorly differentiated lymphocytic lymphoma

This disease has a relatively rapid course and is more difficult to treat. Involvement of extranodal sites is seen frequently and these may be the only sites of disease at presentation (e.g. lymphosarcoma of the stomach). Treatment should include both radiotherapy, for sites of bulky disease, and chemotherapy. A well-tried combination of drugs is cyclophosphamide, vincristine and prednisone, but newer agents such as adriamycin, bleomycin and the nitrosoureas are also useful. Occasionally, the malignant poorly differentiated lymphocytes are seen circulating in the blood. Here the disease may be treated as acute lymphoblastic leukaemia using vincristine and prednisone to achieve remission, followed by prophylactic cranial irradiation with intrathecal chemotherapy or spinal irradiation (see Chapter 9).

Diffuse histiocytic lymphomas

Diffuse histiocytic lymphomas comprise the group of diseases previously covered by the term 'reticulum-cell sarcoma'. A particularly high incidence of this lymphoma is seen in patients receiving immunosuppressive treatment after renal transplantation. The clinical features are as for the other lymphomas and extra nodal involvement (e.g. in bone) is common. Although this disease carries a relatively poor prognosis, prolonged remissions may be obtained, particularly after complete remission has been achieved with combination chemotherapy. The best-tested agents are cyclophosphamide, vincristine and procarbazine, but newer agents, particularly adriamycin, are of value. Radiotherapy is used for areas of previous bulky disease after chemotherapy has achieved a remission.

Burkitt's lymphoma

Burkitt's lymphoma is a separate entity from the other malignant lymphomas and has several unique features. It occurs predominantly in a well-defined geographical region of equatorial Africa where it is confined to warm rainy areas. It is virtually unknown in adjacent arid regions. It is also common in New Guinea, but is seen only sporadically elsewhere in the world. These geographical considerations suggest a possible infectious aetiology and there is now considerable serological evidence associating a herpes virus (Epstein–Barr virus) with this disease. Burkitt's lymphoma is seen principally in children. Pathologically it is characterised by the presence in the lymph nodes of undifferentiated cells arranged diffusely and lacking any marked differentiation towards either the lymphocytic or histiocytic type. Numerous macrophages within the tumour containing ingested cellular debris produce the so-called 'starry-sky' appearance. Enormous facial tumours may be seen in the commonest form of the disease which involves the region of the maxilla or mandible. Any part of the body, however, may be affected and abdominal masses, ascites, retro-orbital tumours and central-nervous-system involvement are common. Burkitt's lymphoma is highly chemosensitive and chemotherapy is the treatment of choice. Cyclophosphamide is particularly effective in inducing remissions but methotrexate, cytosine arabinoside and the vinca-alkaloids are also effective. Cell kinetic studies have shown that this tumour has a growth fraction approaching 100 per cent and this offers an explanation for its remarkable sensitivity to cytotoxic drugs. Central-nervous-system disease is best treated by intrathecal methotrexate or cytosine arabinoside.

Many patients with this disease achieve prolonged remissions after chemotherapy, suggesting cure in many cases. The most favourable outlook is in patients with tumours confined to the facial area, while abdominal and central-nervous involvement carries a poorer prognosis.

CHAPTER ELEVEN

HEAD AND NECK

The malignant tumours classified conventionally as head and neck cancers arise in the upper air and digestive passages (oral cavity, pharynx, larynx, paranasal sinuses, nasopharynx and salivary glands). Other tumours occurring in the head and neck are discussed elsewhere. The majority of malignant tumours arising in the mucosa of the upper air and digestive passages are squamous-cell carcinomas, which characteristically enlarge and invade locally and metastasise to lymph nodes in the neck; distant metastases generally occur very late in the natural history of these diseases.

ORAL CAVITY

Tumours of the oral cavity may arise in the lips, buccal mucosa, floor of mouth, tongue and gums. Certain evidence suggests that excessive use of alcohol and tobacco predisposes to these tumours and prolonged exposure to sunlight may be relevant to the development of cancers of the lip. Leukoplakia (white plaques of hyperkeratosis) with atypia in the buccal cavity is well recognised as a premalignant lesion, but hyperkeratosis without atypia rarely goes on to produce cancers. Squamous-cell carcinomas in the oral cavity are treacherous tumours with a propensity for invasion of adjacent structures such as infiltration of the mandible and the tongue musculature which ultimately affects speech articulation and deglutition.

Massive haemorrhage may result from invasion of blood vessels. A late, but rare, complication is the development of an oro-cutaneous fistula. Clinically, metastases occur in the cervical lymph nodes and dissemination to other sites occurs late; at autopsy a number of cases have demonstrable metastases in the lungs, liver and bones. Death is often due to pneumonia.

Curative treatment is dependent on the precise site and size of the primary tumour and the extent of invasion and dissemination. Small tumours can be eradicated frequently by either radiotherapy or limited surgery, but for more advanced tumours, radical procedures are required and it is thought by some to be expedient to combine surgery and radiotherapy. Operations may be mutilating, but in expert hands and with skilful reconstructive procedures, excellent cosmetic results can sometimes be achieved. Even a poor cosmetic result or residual disability after surgery are preferable to the distress and misery that results from leaving these tumours untreated. Lymphatic metastases should be treated by radical neck dissection, although survival of patients with such involvement is considerably less than if the nodes are unaffected. Studies of adjuvant post-operative chemotherapy are now in progress. Experience with chemotherapy has so far been gained in the advanced disease no longer amenable to surgical treatment or radiotherapy. The most active drug is methotrexate, but bleomycin, vincristine and adriamycin are also of value.

Dental tumours

Tumours arising from the cells concerned with the production of dentine, enamel and cementum (odontoblasts, ameloblasts and cemento-blasts respectively) are rare. Generally, they are benign, but on rare occasions may become malignant. Dental tumours can usually be treated successfully by either excision or curretage, and the prognosis is excellent although sometimes there is a tendency to local recurrence.

PHARYNX

Conventionally the pharynx is divided into three regions, naso-pharynx, oropharynx (including the pillars of the fauces and tonsils) and hypopharynx (including the posterior tongue, pyriform fossae and the post-cricoid area).

Nasopharynx

Nasopharyngeal cancer is uncommon in Europe and North America. It occurs more frequently in Africa and South-East Asia, where patients with these tumours often have circulating antibodies to Burkitt lymphoma cells, suggesting an aetiological relationship between these two cancers. Nasopharyngeal tumours are squamous-cell carcinomas, but lymphocytic infiltration may be considerable and these tumours have been named lymphoepitheliomas. These tumours invade locally and involvement of the base of skull, with cranial nerve palsies, nasal obstruction and haemorrhage are common. They may also present as serous otitis media or with lymphatic metastases. Nasopharyngeal carcinoma is diagnosed at rhinoscopy, and the diagnosis confirmed under general anaesthesia when a biopsy is taken. This should be accompanied by careful radiological examination to determine the precise extent of the tumour. The usual treatment is radiotherapy to the primary tumour and regional lymph nodes, but lymph-node metastases are usefully treated by radical neck dissection when the primary is under control and overt metastases are still present.

Oropharynx

Tumours of the oropharynx tend to be rather more poorly dif-ferentiated squamous-cell carcinomas than those arising in the mouth and larynx, and there is a high incidence of cervical lymph-node metastases at the time of presentation. Sometimes, first presentation is due to cervical lymph-node masses, a search having to be made for the primary site.

Overall, the prognosis for oropharyngeal tumours is poor, approximately one third of patients surviving 5 years. Treatment varies between different centres, but generally the preferred approach is radiotherapy, surgery being reserved for failed radiotherapy, or, on occasions, as part of a combined plan. Radical neck dissection is often appropriate for metastases in cervical lymph nodes.

Hypopharynx

Cancers of the hypopharynx may be associated with heavy smoking and also with iron-deficiency anaemia in women (Plummer–Vinson syndrome). Clinically, these tumours lead to disorders of swallowing and extension to the larynx may interfere with speech. They are frequently advanced at the time of presentation, often with cervical lymph-node metastases. Hypopharyngeal tumours can generally be seen at indirect laryngoscopy, and diagnosis is confirmed by biopsy taken at direct laryngoscopy. Surgical procedures are occasionally curative and offer the patient the prospect of being able to swallow again. For operable tumours, radiotherapy may be used, but the most appropriate treatment depends on the site and extent of the tumour and the presence or absence of metastases. The prognosis is generally very poor.

LARYNX

Carcinoma of the larynx is confined almost entirely to heavy smokers. If situated on the vocal cords, it can be detected when small and before invasion has occurred, owing to the striking voice changes that are produced. Supra- and sub-glottic tumours, however, are not usually detected at such an early stage. Even more than cancer of the vocal cord, they invade locally to affect the laryngeal musculature and may enlarge sufficiently to cause obstruction to the airway. Lymph-node metastases from laryngeal carcinomas occur in the deep cervical and paratracheal group and then subsequently in cervical lymph nodes. Laryngeal tumours can usually be seen by indirect laryngoscopy and tomograms are helpful in indicating their extent. Diagnosis is by biopsy taken at direct laryngoscopy.

Small tumours confined to the vocal cords are generally curable by radiotherapy, but for more extensive tumours, cure usually requires total laryngectomy. Partial supra-glottic laryngectomy may be feasible for limited tumours of the supra-glottis. For more advanced tumours some believe that it is expedient to combine both surgery and radiotherapy. After laryngectomy, about 40 per cent of patients can be taught to develop an oesophageal voice, but when this cannot be achieved, various mechanical and electronic devices are available to help restore speech.

For laryngeal carcinomas situated in the centre of a mobile vocal cord, cure rates of 90 per cent are quoted. However, overall five-year survival rate for localised laryngeal cancers is about 60 per cent and this drops to

30 per cent when regional lymph-node involvement is present. The role of adjuvant chemotherapy is now being investigated.

PARANASAL SINUSES

The majority of paranasal-sinus cancers are again squamous-cell carcinomas, but, occasionally, adenocarcinomas and mesenchymal tumours arise. Most of these tumours occur in the maxillary sinus, tumours of the ethmoid being uncommon and sphenoid and frontal sinuses being very rare. They are often advanced at diagnosis, the presenting symptoms being due to extension into the orbit or cheek, cranial nerve involvement or the development of a palatal mass. Only occasionally are these tumours detected at an early stage when attention may be drawn to them by the occurrence of nasal bleeding.

Tomograms are of value in defining the extent of these tumours and exploration of the antrum may be necessary for biopsy. Usually combined therapy is prescribed, radiotherapy preceding surgery, which consists of partial or total maxillectomy with or without orbital enucleation. The overall 5-year survival for paranasal sinus cancer is only 20–30 per cent.

SALIVARY GLANDS

The majority of tumours arising in the salivary glands are benign, although these have a tendency to recur locally unless adequate excision with careful dissection of the facial nerve is performed. Malignant salivary-gland tumours usually occur in the parotid or sub-mandibular glands and only uncommonly in the sub-lingual gland. Parotid tumours which are deeply situated may present as pharyngeal swellings with no external mass being evident. The histology of salivary-gland malignant tumours varies considerably, but broadly speaking can be divided into high- and low-grade tumours.

Malignant salivary-gland tumours may present as painful facial swellings which are irregular, hard, and often fixed to skin. Parotid tumours with invasion of the facial nerve lead to facial paralysis. Local invasion may involve the middle ear and the base of the skull with metastases to the regional lymph nodes. Distant metastases also occur with adenoid cystic carcinomas, in which pulmonary metastases may remain asymptomatic for many years.

If technically possible, the treatment of choice is excision of the tumour with radical neck dissection, if the cervical nodes are involved; for infiltrating parotid tumours the facial nerve often has to be sacrificed. Radiotherapy is reserved generally for inoperable cases. Because of the likelihood of adenoid cystic carcinomas spreading in the cephalad direction it is advisable to give post-operative radiotherapy, the upper level of the treatment field being the base of skull. The prognosis is very variable, depending on the site and histology of the tumour.

CHAPTER TWELVE

SKIN

This chapter includes an account of pre-malignant conditions of the skin, primary tumours of the skin and dermatological manifestations of malignant disease elsewhere.

PRE-MALIGNANT CONDITIONS

Malignant change in the skin is seen more often with increasing age and is unusual under the age of 40. Exposure to sunlight is an important and common cause of malignant change in the skin of white people who lack the protective properties conferred by melanin in coloured races. White people living in parts of Australia, Africa, Central America and Asia are particularly prone to skin cancer. Atrophy of the normal skin occurs on prolonged exposure to sunlight and later solar keratoses appear which may become epitheliomas. Prolonged exposure of the skin to high doses of X-rays causes atrophy and telangiectasia with eventual malignant change. This used to occur frequently among medical personnel who were concerned with the early use of X-ray apparatus. Workers who handle tar, pitch, bitumen and mineral oils may develop keratoses or warts and later epitheliomas, usually occurring on the exposed skin, but one well-known example is the epithelioma of the scrotum caused by prolonged contact with mineral oil soaking into trousers from machinery. Arsenic compounds ingested in the past in various medicines or applied to the skin accidentally but repeatedly as sheep-dip or fungicides may cause changes many years later. These include the appearance of Bowen's disease (intra-epidermal carcinoma). Finally, old ulcerated scars due to burns or leukoplakia, particularly of the vulva and anus, may undergo malignant change.

MALIGNANT TUMOURS

Basal cell carcinoma (rodent ulcer)

This is the commonest malignant condition of the skin. It occurs during or after middle age and usually involves the forehead, eyelids, cheeks and nose. White-skinned people exposed to sunlight are particularly susceptible.

Pathology

The lesion begins as a small pearly nodule which enlarges slowly over the course of months and eventually ulcerates, producing the characteristic rolled edge of the rodent ulcer. It can invade deep structures including bone and cartilage. Metastasis is extremely rare. Numerous darkly stained basal cells arising in the epidermis give a characteristic histological appearance.

Diagnosis

The lesion is usually easily recognised clinically but occasionally it may be pigmented and then confused with a melanoma. Proof of the diagnosis is obtained by histological examination.

Treatment

Surgical excision of the lesion produces a cure rate of between 90 and 95 per cent. This is the most satisfactory method of treatment but with large lesions or those at certain sites such as the eyelids, or when patients are very frail, radiotherapy produces equally good results. With large lesions or when bone or cartilage are involved, as a result of deep invasion, excision may need to be followed by reconstructive plastic surgery.

Squamous-cell carcinoma (epitheliomas)

These tumours are less common than basal-cell carcinomas and usually arise in previously damaged skin.

Clinical features

There is usually shallow ulceration with an irregular outline and a raised edge. The lesion bleeds easily.

Pathology

There are varying grades of malignancy, depending upon the degree of differentiation of the proliferating epidermal cells and the extent of invasion of the dermis. This may vary from well-differentiated cells with keratinisation to undifferentiated spindle-shaped cells without keratinisation. Metastasis is relatively uncommon but occurs initially to the regional lymph nodes and is more likely to occur with tumours at mucocutaneous junctions.

Diagnosis

Solar keratoses resemble early epitheliomata and indeed are liable to become malignant. Kerato-acanthoma may resemble a well-differentiated epithelioma. Histological examination confirms diagnosis.

Treatment

Excision of the primary lesion leads to a cure rate of 75 to 80 per cent, but it depends upon the maturity of the cell type and the presence of lymph-node metastases. The less differentiated tumours tend to recur and metastasise early. Radiotherapy is also effective and should be used when surgical excision is incomplete or where the site of the tumour precludes its removal.

Bowen's disease (intra-epidermal carcinoma)

This condition is uncommon. It comprises erythematous plaques which are well defined and which grow slowly. They are mainly found on the trunk and during the course of several years extend up to several centimetres in length. Spread is along the epidermal plain but in time invasion takes place and the lesions then behave as squamous-cell carcinomas.

Differential diagnosis

A solitary lesion may be very similar to that of psoriasis but the plaques tend to persist and when a history of exposure to arsenic over a prolonged period is obtained, this should suggest the diagnosis: biopsy is essential to establish this.

Treatment

The lesions are not radiosensitive, and the best treatment is excision.

Paget's disease of the nipple (see Chapter 8)

Malignant melanoma

Most fair-skinned people have numerous pigmented moles and malignant change is extremely rare. Malignant melanoma accounts for approximately 1 per cent of all cancers and has a peak incidence between 50 and 60 years.

Pathology

Malignant melanoma is a tumour of the melanocytes usually situated in the basal layer of the epidermis. Spread is by direct extension along fascial planes, by embolism in lymphatic or blood vessels or as intra-epithelial satellites. Repeated trauma of a benign junctional mole may produce malignant change.

Clinical features

There are three types of malignant melanoma which are recognisable clinically.

1 **Lentigo maligna or Hutchinson's freckle.**
This almost always occurs in the elderly and the mean age is about 70 years. It is found on the face and is a flat area of grey-black discolouration. It remains impalpable but increases in area very slowly and after approximately twenty years tends to develop nodular changes.

2 **Superficial spreading melanoma.**
This is the most common type of tumour and occurs usually on the face, head and neck, soles of the feet, and near or under the nails. A pre-existing brown or black mole usually undergoes malignant changes although melanomas can arise *de novo*. Typically, however, there is an increase in size with irregular change in or loss or spread of pigment. In addition, variation in colour, outline, ulceration, bleeding or the presence of inflammation are all signs of malignant change, as are enlarged regional lymph nodes.

3 **Nodular melanoma.**
This is the most malignant form which shows little lateral growth and consists of a nodule which is usually black, purple or dark brown in colour.

Both superficial spreading melanoma and nodular melanoma are found in younger patients than in those with lentigo maligna and the mean age is in the late forties or early fifties, but the range is wide. Amelanotic melanomas do not contain pigment, are more difficult to recognise clinically, but are uncommon. Regional lymph nodes may be enlarged due to metastatic spread, and wide dissemination ultimately occurs with metastases found most often in the skin, liver, brain and lungs.

Investigations

The single most important investigation is biopsy, which is essential to establish the diagnosis. The lesion should also be measured and the presence or absence of underlying fixation noted. The size of the lesion and the degree of penetration into the lower levels of the skin are the most important factors which determine survival. Blood counts, liver scan, chest radiography and radiographs of local structures where any fixation is suspected are important in assessing whether metastatic spread has occurred. Bone scans should be undertaken to exclude the presence of skeletal metastases.

Treatment

Surgery offers the best chance of cure and radical local excision with, if necessary, a skin graft is the treatment of choice for the primary tumour. Melanomas less than 2 cm in diameter and confined to the epidermis only, if adequately treated, are associated with an 80 per cent 5-year survival. As the tumour size increases and the degree of penetration into the skin is deeper, so the prognosis becomes increasingly poor. Resection of regional lymph nodes is usually undertaken in continuity when the position of the primary tumour allows this, but in the case of a limb this is often not possible. Radiotherapy is of limited value in the treatment of melanomas but some workers have claimed improved results with post-operative irradiation. This form of treatment can be useful for palliation of isolated lesions or bone pain.

Chemotherapy is undergoing active investigation and some drugs appear to be producing significant benefit. Decarbazine is capable of producing objective regression of the tumour in about 20 per cent of patients, while alkylating agents, nitrosoureas, vincristine and procarbazine are occasionally of value. Better results are being claimed with combinations. As spontaneous general or local regressions are sometimes observed in malignant melanomas, there has been considerable interest in immunological aspects of this tumour. Attempts to modify the course of the disease with systemic or intra-lesional injections of B.C.G. and the use of vaccines, prepared from melanoma cells, either alone or combined with systemic chemotherapy, have been studied, but in well-controlled studies the results have so far been disappointing.

Metastases

Metastases from tumours elsewhere are frequently found in the skin, particularly from cancers of the breast, bronchus and gastro-intestinal tract. When they are limited in number and extent they may be excised or irradiated, otherwise they may respond to systemic therapy.

Mycosis fungoides

This rare cutaneous syndrome, despite its name, is not associated with a fungal infection, but is an infiltration of the skin histologically resembling a malignant lymphoma. Initially, there are erythematous scaly plaques which cause itching. These increase in size, become nodular and later undergo ulceration. The areas may be very extensive and the patient usually succumbs from generalised lymphoma. Local treatment with radiotherapy is effective where the lesions are small enough and chemotherapy is moderately effective, the most useful drugs being cyclophosphamide, vincristine and prednisolone.

SKIN MANIFESTATIONS OF MALIGNANT DISEASE ELSEWHERE

Acanthosis Nigricans

This consists of abnormal pigmentation and hypertrophy of the skin in the hands, feet and flexures (particularly the axillae and groins). Warty areas develop which become fissured. This condition is most often found in association with carcinoma of the stomach.

Dermatomyositis

In this condition there are inflammatory changes in the skin, muscle and blood vessels producing oedema, especially around the eyes, and erythema, particularly in areas where the muscles are painful and weak, usually around the shoulder and hip girdles. Areas of skin exposed to the light are also affected and, initially, the erythema has a violet appearance later becoming brown in colour. Biopsy of the skin and muscle reveals inflammatory cells infiltrating the connective tissue and around the blood vessels. Muscle enzymes (creatine phosphokinase and lactic dehydrogenase) in the blood are elevated. In adults with this condition up to 50 per cent are subsequently found to have an underlying neoplasm which is most commonly in the lung.

Other skin eruptions

There are numerous other skin conditions associated with underlying malignant disease but which do not have the above specific features. Any unusual skin eruption occurring after the age of 40 should be regarded with suspicion and may indicate an underlying neoplasm. There are, however, some more common associations such as generalised pruritus which occurs in Hodgkin's disease and less often a generalised exfoliative dermatitis may precede other lymphomas. Erythema with an annular distribution and accompanied by superficial necrosis of the skin is sometimes seen with carcinoma of the pancreas. Urticaria, pemphigoid and lesions resembling erythema multiforme are also seen occasionally with occult neoplasms. Herpes zoster sometimes occurs in a dermatome adjacent to a metastatic deposit in the spine, but, apart from this, there is a high incidence of shingles in patients with malignant disease, particularly lymphomas, probably due to associated suppressed immunity.

CHAPTER THIRTEEN

URINARY TRACT

This chapter gives an account of malignant tumours of the kidney, ureter and bladder. Tumours of the renal parenchyma have special characteristics but those of the renal pelvis share with tumours of the ureter and bladder similar features since the epithelium is the same and it is exposed to identical carcinogens. Wilms' tumour (nephroblastoma) is described in Chapter 19.

THE KIDNEY

The most common tumour of the kidney is the hypernephroma, also known as renal-cell carcinoma or renal adenocarcinoma, which comprises 80 per cent of all kidney tumours. Transitional-cell carcinomas and squamous-cell carcinomas of the renal pelvis account for the remainder of primary kidney tumours and are histologically similar to those of the ureter and bladder. Hypernephroma occurs twice as often in men as in women and the average age at diagnosis is 55–60. Occasionally this tumour may be multiple or bilateral. Nothing is known about its cause.

Pathology

Hypernephroma may grow slowly and remain quiescent for a long time. Metastases usually spread in the blood stream to the liver, lungs, brain and bones but other sites may be involved, including the opposite kidney. Lymph nodes in the region of the pedicle are invaded and spread may take place more widely by this route. The kidney is a natural source of erythropoietin and in a small proportion of renal tumours excessive amounts of this substance are produced, leading to erythrocytosis.

Clinical features

Common symptoms of a kidney tumour are haematuria and, less often, pain in the renal region. Sometimes the diagnosis is made when a mass is felt during routine examination, but many patients present with a variety of features unrelated to the urinary tract. Fever occurs often and may be the presenting symptom, while a small proportion have hypertension, anaemia or hypercalcaemia. Examination may reveal a mass in the flank and if the tumour has spread there may be signs of inferior vena caval obstruction. Because of the unusual ways in which this tumour presents, there is often a long delay between the initial symptoms and diagnosis; it is, therefore, important to remember the possibility of this tumour in a patient with obscure symptoms.

Investigations

Examination of the urine may show red blood cells. The most important and useful investigations are radiological. An enlarged kidney may be seen in a plain abdominal X-ray, but intravenous urography combined with tomography provides the best information. A space occupying lesion in the kidney leads to stretched, deformed and elongated calyces, usually at one or other pole, but if there has been extensive invasion of the kidney substance or if the renal vein has become occluded there may be no excretion on that side. Angiography with selective filling of renal arteries allows confident diagnosis to be made in almost every instance because of the characteristic new vessels produced by the tumour. It may also be possible at the same time to detect metastases in the liver by injecting dye into the coeliac axis.

Very often there is doubt after intravenous urography as to whether a lesion is a cyst or a tumour, but the use of ultra-sonography distinguishes between them. Precise recognition of a cyst is possible by needle aspiration and the introduction of an opaque medium. Venography may be necessary to determine whether a tumour has spread to involve the inferior vena cava or renal vein, since this will affect the feasibility of surgery. Other investigations include a chest X-ray, perhaps with tomography, and a bone scan to detect metastases. Liver involvement is suggested by abnormal liver-function tests and estimation of plasma calcium is necessary together with a full blood count.

Treatment

When no metastases are demonstrable, the most effective treatment is a radical nephrectomy including removal of perinephric fat, the adrenal gland, and the lymphatics from the diaphragm to the aortic bifurcation. When distant metastases are present a simple nephrectomy will be necessary in most cases to relieve haematuria and pain. In the case of bilateral tumours it is sometimes possible to treat these by performing either partial nephrectomy on both sides or bilateral nephrectomy, and maintaining life by means of intermittent haemodialysis. Radiotherapy is usually reserved for post-operative treatment when it has not been possible to remove the whole tumour, but these tumours are relatively radio-resistant.

Chemotherapy has been attempted and drugs used have included vinblastine, 6-mercaptopurine and hydroxyurea but tumour regression is unusual, incomplete and temporary. Many patients have also been treated with medroxyprogesterone because of reported regression following such treatment, but its value is uncertain. Similarly regression of metastases has occurred after nephrectomy but this is also an uncommon occurrence and should not be anticipated.

CARCINOMA OF THE RENAL PELVIS

This constitutes about 14 per cent of kidney tumours and comprises transitional-cell carcinomas, which are histologically similar to those of the ureter and bladder, and the less common squamous-cell carcinomas which follow chronic infection and calculus formation and consequent metaplasia of transitional epithelium. The latter tumours, since infection is usually present, are difficult to diagnose and, therefore, often treated late, with a poor prognosis. Treatment consists of resection of the kidney and adjacent ureter. Radiotherapy and chemotherapy are ineffective.

The transitional-cell carcinoma of the renal pelvis tends to affect males over the age of 50 and presents with haematuria and ureteric colic. The intravenous urogram shows irregular filling defects in the renal pelvis and in the ureter, since there is a tendency for these tumours to be multicentric. Treatment consists of removal of the kidney, ureter and part of the bladder surrounding the ureteric orifice. Regular inspection of the bladder should follow such treatment to detect recurrent disease at that site. The results of treatment of transitional-cell carcinoma are better than for squamous carcinoma, since the former are usually recognised earlier.

CARCINOMA OF THE BLADDER

Transitional-cell carcinoma is the commonest tumour of the bladder in the United Kingdom, Europe and North America when it forms part of a generalised urothelial disease involving the renal pelvis, ureter and bladder. These areas are all in contact with urine and certain agents excreted by the kidneys are known to be carcinogenic. Although in individual cases the cause of carcinoma of the bladder is usually not known, there is a very strong association between this disease and exposure to certain industrial chemicals, notably the aromatic amines which are used in the dyestuffs and rubber industries. Beta-naphthylamine is the most powerful carcinogen encountered in these conditions, followed by alpha-naphthylamine and benzidine. These substances, which were used widely in industry, were banned in the United Kingdom in 1976 but cases are still appearing where exposure occurred many years before. Other chemicals are also known to be carcinogenic and these include aniline and ortho-tolidine. It is also known that there is a higher incidence of bladder cancer amongst smokers and those who drink large quantities of coffee. It is worth noting that benzidine was formerly used for the detection of occult blood in the faeces by doctors, nurses or technicians and that ortho-tolidine is still used to test the chlorine content of water in swimming pools.

Squamous-cell carcinoma of the bladder has a different aetiology. It is closely associated with schistosomiasis and there is a lesser association with chronic bladder infection and calculi. *S.haematobium*, which is endemic in several parts of the world, but notably in the rural areas of Egypt, is the organism associated with bladder cancer and this tumour is common in these areas.

Pathology

Carcinoma of the bladder varies from lesions which resemble benign polyps and which have a very slow recurring course over many years, to tumours which are deeply invasive at an early stage with rapid and aggressive growth, a short duration and early death. The histological appearance of the tumour closely mirrors the anatomical staging and well-differentiated tumours tend to be superficial and confined to the bladder, whereas undifferentiated tumours show invasive features with spread to the neighbouring pelvic structures, lymph nodes and more distant metastases, particularly in the liver, lung and bones.

Clinical features

Haematuria, which is usually painless, is the commonest presenting symptom. It may be intermittent and if ignored, leads to a delay in the diagnosis. Other symptoms include dysuria with frequency, and sometimes urinary obstruction. Physical examination is usually unhelpful but occasionally rectal examination may reveal fixation or lateral extension of a bladder tumour.

Investigations

Examination of the urine shows in most instances microscopic haematuria and cytological examination may show malignant cells. This is a screening procedure used in industry which allows the detection of early lesions in people who are at risk. In the case of patients suspected of schistosomiasis the examination of a urine specimen for the ova of schistosoma is helpful.

Intravenous urography is an important investigation which may show lesions in the ureters and indicate whether they are patent or not as well as showing the bladder outline and demonstrating the presence of filling defects. A chest radiograph is necessary to exclude pulmonary metastases and either a bone scan or skeletal radiographs should be undertaken when appropriate, but particularly if there is bone pain. Lymphography is sometimes helpful to assess whether lymph-node involvement has occurred. The most important investigation is cystoscopy to inspect the tumour, show its exact site and size, and whether or not it is multicentric. Biopsy of the lesion is essential and small lesions may be completely resected. At cystoscopy a bimanual examination under anaesthetic is necessary to feel the state of the pelvic organs to assess the extent of disease. The most important factor in predicting the prognosis is the depth of penetration into the bladder wall.

Treatment

Superficial bladder carcinoma is usually managed by resection and local diathermy which in the great majority of cases is achieved at cystoscopy. About 60 per cent of such patients have recurrent disease and careful follow-up is essential. The high incidence of recurrence may be due to residual tumour after resection or continued exposure to a carcinogen in the urine. Sometimes a large superficial lesion in a difficult site can only be satisfactorily treated by partial cystectomy. When there are small, multiple superficial lesions some workers believe that a reduction in the rate of recurrence can be achieved by instilling thiotepa into the bladder about three weeks after endoscopic resection or fulguration. This is done through a urinary catheter and is repeated at intervals initially of a week and then a month. An alternative agent with similar effects is ethoglucid. The use of external or intra-cavity radiation in these circumstances has not proved particularly effective.

The optimal treatment of invasive lesions is uncertain and approaches include radical radiotherapy, surgery or a combination of the two. Radical surgery includes total cystectomy with removal of the pelvic nodes, the prostate and seminal vesicles with the provision of an ileal conduit diverting urine to the abdominal wall for collection in a bag. This is justified only if the patient has an otherwise reasonable life expectation, is fit for such surgery and if there is no evidence of metastatic disease outside the bladder. Radical radiotherapy may also be used when surgical means have failed to control recurrent disease. Palliative treatment is given to control pain and haematuria.

Although local chemotherapy has proved useful in the management of multiple superficial lesions, it has so far been disappointing in the management of large lesions. Several agents have been used topically, including 5-fluorouracil and actinomycin D, but the results have been generally poor. Systemic chemotherapy has not so far been effective, but recent results using newer agents in combination, such as Adriamycin, methotrexate and cis-platinum, show some promise.

The prognosis of patients with superficial cancers treated by careful endoscopic resection or fulguration is good, with a 5-year survival rate approaching 80 per cent. Invasive carcinoma of the bladder has a worse prognosis but the 5-year survival rate has improved since the use of pre-operative radiotherapy followed by total cystectomy, and now approaches 50 per cent.

CHAPTER FOURTEEN

THE MALE REPRODUCTIVE SYSTEM

PROSTATE GLAND

Carcinoma of the prostate is the commonest tumour in men over the age of 60 and the median age of incidence is 70 years.

The incidence shows considerable geographical variation and increases with each decade over 50 years. At autopsy, histological evidence of carcinoma of the prostate is found more often than the clinical disease is diagnosed.

Pathology

Virtually all carcinomas of the prostate are adenocarcinomas and although most are well differentiated, the degree of differentiation has an important influence upon the prognosis. Spread is mainly by local extension into the bladder, but lymph nodes are often involved in the pelvis and occasionally the inguinal region. Spread through the blood stream occurs commonly, giving rise to metastases in bones and, less often, other organs. Metastases to bone characteristically excite an osteosclerotic reaction.

Clinical features

A small carcinoma of the prostate can occasionally be detected as a nodule felt on rectal examination without any history of prostatic disease. Symptoms are usually those of urethral obstruction, with dribbling, a poor stream and, ultimately, acute retention. Unlike benign prostatic hypertrophy the history is short and rapidly progressive. Cystitis may occur but bleeding is uncommon. Occasionally a carcinoma of the prostate is discovered when the gland is removed for apparent benign hypertrophy. Advanced disease with metastases presents as bone pain often in the spine and pelvis or sciatica. Renal failure may occur due to obstruction to the bladder neck or there may be anaemia due to marrow invasion.

On rectal examination there is nodular prostatic enlargement which feels hard and inguinal lymph nodes may sometimes be involved.

Investigations

The diagnosis can be established by needle biopsy of the prostate, either through the trans-rectal approach or the perineum. Otherwise the diagnosis is made after trans-urethral resection. An intravenous urogram is necessary and will reveal, if present, ureteric obstruction or deformity of the bladder outline. A bone scan or radiological skeletal survey should be performed in order to detect the presence of metastases, which are found most often in the pelvis or vertebrae, and in the great majority of cases are sclerotic, but there may be a combination of osteoblastic and lytic lesions; isolated lytic lesions are rare. Chest radiography rarely shows pulmonary metastases but lymphography should be undertaken to assess lymph-node involvement in the abdomen and pelvis. Examination of the blood may show a leuko-erythroblastic anaemia due to marrow invasion. The acid and alkaline phosphatases are raised in about 75 per cent of cases when there are bone metastases, but it is important to take blood for estimation of the acid phosphatase either before rectal examination or several hours afterwards, since this alone can increase the level.

Treatment

After the exclusion of metastatic disease, radiotherapy to the prostate and pelvic node fields is the treatment usually undertaken. Unlike radical surgical treatment (removal of the prostate, seminal vesicles and a cuff of bladder neck) this preserves sexual function and does not lead to incontinence. Some centres simply use oestrogens alone as primary treatment.

In the case of advanced disease, regressions usually follow suppression of testosterone activity. Treatment consists of either bilateral orchidectomy or the administration of oestrogens. This may be combined with a transurethral resection if there is urinary obstruction. Symptoms are relieved in about 90 per cent of patients with this form of treatment. Stilboestrol in a dose of 1–5 mg daily is usually sufficient, but large intravenous doses of fosfestrol may sometimes relieve symptoms due to relapse.

Radiotherapy to metastatic lesions is valuable to relieve symptoms, and radioactive phosphorus (^{32}P) has also been used effectively. Corticosteroids in the form of prednisolone are sometimes helpful for relief and about 10 per cent of patients respond to hypophysectomy. Chemotherapy is usually disappointing, although cyclophosphamide has been used with some benefit and other agents are occasionally moderately successful.

TESTIS

Tumours of the testis constitute 1–2 per cent of cancers in males and occur in the 20–40 age group, the mean age being 32 years. The cause is unknown but there is a much higher incidence in undescended testes, particularly if sited within the abdomen.

Pathology

There is a wide variety of histological types and the nomenclature is confusing since terminology is variable. A simplified classification of testicular tumours is given in Table 14.1.

TABLE 14.1   Tumours of the testis

U.K.	U.S.A.
Seminoma	Seminoma
Differentiated teratoma	Teratoma
Malignant teratoma	
Intermediate type	Teratocarcinoma
Anaplastic	Embryonal carcinoma
Trophoblastic	Choriocarcinoma
Combined tumours	Combined tumours
Interstitial-cell tumours	Interstitial-cell tumours

Spread occurs by direct extension into the epidydimis and in the lymphatics to the para-aortic then, retrogradely, to the ipsilateral iliac lymph nodes. Blood-stream spread gives rise to pulmonary metastases.

Clinical features

Tumours of the testis usually present as a painless swelling which on examination is found to be hard, solid and non-tender. Although the tumour cannot be transilluminated, a secondary hydrocoele may form. Symptoms due to metastatic disease include weight loss, fatigue and back pain due to involved retroperitoneal nodes. Pulmonary metastases may give rise to breathlessness, cough and occasionally haemoptysis.

Investigations

Any testicular mass should be explored surgically by the inguinal route, the testis and cord being removed. In the case of a malignant tumour a chest radiograph may show pulmonary metastases, delineated more clearly by whole-lung tomography. Lymphography should be undertaken to assess lymphatic involvement and intravenous urography gives information about renal function and the presence of ureteric displacement. The blood or urine should be examined for alpha fetoprotein since elevated levels are usually found with malignant teratomas. Chorionic gonadotrophin and placental lactogen may be detectable with trophoblastic tumours.

Staging

Before considering treatment of these tumours it is useful to stage the extent of disease. A simple and convenient method is as follows:

Stage I   tumour confined to the testis;
Stage II   involvement of para-aortic and/or ipsilateral iliac lymph nodes but not nodes above the diaphragm;

Stage III   involvement of lymph nodes above the diaphragm but not extra-nodal structures;

Stage IV   extra-lymphatic dissemination (usually pulmonary).

Although there is a good correlation between tumour staging and prognosis, tumour bulk is also important. For example, massive Stage II disease carries a worse prognosis than Stage IV disease when only a solitary pulmonary metastasis is present.

Treatment

After orchidectomy, during the investigation of these tumours, subsequent treatment depends upon the histological type and staging.

Seminoma. This is an extremely radiosensitive tumour and in Stage I disease it is essential to follow orchidectomy by radiotherapy to the para-aortic and ipsilateral iliac lymph nodes. The prognosis of Stage I seminomas treated this way is excellent, with a 5-year survival of at least 85–90 per cent. In Stage II disease the field should be extended to include the mediastinum and left supraclavicular fossa. This extended radiotherapy field should also be used in the treatment of Stage III seminomas and the use of adjuvant chemotherapy in these circumstances is being evaluated. Seminomas are sensitive to alkylating agents and these are used to treat Stage IV disease.

Malignant teratoma. These are more aggressive tumours, often widespread at diagnosis and less responsive to treatment than seminomas. The current approach to the treatment of malignant teratomas is similar to that of seminomas with regard to radiotherapy after orchidectomy. However, the 5-year survival for localised disease is only about 50 per cent.

A variety of cytotoxic drugs, including vinblastine, methotrexate, actinomycin D, chlorambucil and mithramycin, are sometimes of value in inducing regression of Stage IV disease, and some of these drugs have been used effectively in combinations. These agents have been more effective in palliating anaplastic malignant teratomas, the intermediate and trophoblastic types being relatively resistant. This contrasts with the marked chemosensitivity of trophoblastic tumours in women (Chapter 15). Recently, further progress has been made in the chemotherapy of teratomas by combining high doses of vinblastine and bleomycin. Although this combination can be extremely toxic, a considerable number of regressions can be achieved, notably in the previously resistant intermediate tumours. Cis-platinum has also been introduced and is proving to be an effective drug. However, there is a high incidence of pulmonary recurrence after successful chemotherapy, and because of this organ-specificity of metastatic disease, the use of pulmonary irradiation, after complete regression has been induced by chemotherapy, is being assessed in some centres. In bulky Stage II disease, it is possible that chemotherapy before radiotherapy, to reduce tumour size, may improve results of treatment.

It is probable that the cure rate of malignant teratomas will have been shown to have improved in the near future, and treatment planning should be facilitated by monitoring tumour-associated products, such as alpha feto-protein, to detect residual tumour after complete regression has been attained clinically.

PENIS

Tumours of the penis are invariably squamous-cell carcinomas which arise on the glans, the sulcus or on the prepuce as either nodules or infiltrating ulcers. There is a wide geographical variation with a relatively low incidence in Europe but a much higher one in Asia, particularly amongst the Chinese. The condition is usually found in the 40–70 age group and it is seen more commonly in uncircumcised men, particularly when living conditions are bad and hygiene is poor.

Spread of the tumour takes place through lymphatic vessels to the deep and superficial inguinal nodes. Inguinal metastases may occur early but more widespread dissemination is usually very late. The diagnosis is usually obvious on inspection of the lesion but biopsy is essential for proof.

Small early lesions may be treated either by radiotherapy or surgical excision with equally good results, most of the penis thereby being preserved. More advanced tumours require radical surgery and if inguinal lymph nodes are involved they should be included in the dissection. When the tumour is confined to the penis the prognosis is good, the 5-year survival approaching 90 per cent. However, for undifferentiated tumours with advanced local spread of lymph-node involvement, survival falls to less than 50 per cent at 5 years.

CHAPTER FIFTEEN

FEMALE REPRODUCTIVE SYSTEM

Tumours of the female reproductive organs account for about a quarter of malignant tumours in women. This chapter covers malignant tumours of the ovaries, body of the uterus, the cervix uteri, vagina, vulva and choriocarcinoma.

OVARY

Primary tumours of the ovary are the third most common cancer of the female genital tract but account for most deaths from this cause. They are more common in better nourished women, higher social groups, the 40–60 year age group, single or infertile women and in Western countries. The number of deaths per annum in England and Wales from ovarian cancer is increasing. About 15–20 per cent of malignant ovarian tumours are metastases.

Pathology

Primary tumours of the ovary comprise a mixed variety of pathological entities. They may be cystic and, of these, the most common are mucinous or serous cystadenocarcinoma, or they may be solid, the adenocarcinoma being the commonest of this type. Other tumours are the solid malignant teratoma and the relatively uncommon, functionally active (sex-cell) tumours. Among these feminisation occurs with the theca granulosa-cell tumours and virilisation with an arrhenoblastoma. Even rarer is the dysgerminoma which is histologically similar to a seminoma. Metastatic disease in the ovaries is encountered frequently from other tumours of the genital tract and from primary cancers of the stomach, bowel, breast and kidney.

Clinical features

Symptoms are usually absent until the disease is well advanced. Even then the patient may complain only of ill-defined symptoms such as malaise or abdominal discomfort. Pain is not a common feature. Examination may reveal a mass in the pelvis or abdomen although advanced cases may present with ascites or symptoms referable to metastases. Malignant, as opposed to benign, ovarian tumours are often bilateral and accompanied by ascites. Other clinical features of the tumour include rapid growth, firm consistency, immobility and nodules in the pouch of Douglas. Evidence of hormonal disturbance is unusual except for the precocious puberty found in young girls with granulosa-cell tumours and masculinisation which is sometimes found with arrhenoblastomas.

Investigations

Cytological examination of the contents of the pouch of Douglas acquired at endoscopy has been undertaken by some investigators, but it is a difficult procedure and the results are uncertain. Laparotomy is required to make the diagnosis with certainty and to assess the extent of the disease. Other important investigations include a chest radiograph and an ultrasound examination. In certain circumstances it may be useful to perform lymphography and a liver scan.

Treatment

Surgery offers the best chance of cure or long-term remission with carcinoma of the ovary and the results depend very much upon the extent at the time of diagnosis and the histological type. Removal of both ovaries (salpingo-oophorectomy) and a total hysterectomy is necessary even if only one ovary is apparently involved. When the tumour has spread beyond the ovary, as much of the tumour should be removed as is feasible and this may include the omentum. Most surgeons advocate removal of the omentum even if not apparently involved, in order to reduce the risk of subsequent peritoneal metastases. Although many ovarian tumours are relatively radio-resistant, post-operative pelvic irradiation is often given and may be extended to include the whole abdomen to destroy occult metastases.

Chemotherapy for more advanced ovarian tumours and, in particular, those which are not completely removed at operation, can lead to remission in 30 to 50 per cent of cases with benefit sometimes lasting for years. The most effective drugs are alkylating agents, of which chlorambucil has been used most often, although cyclophosphamide and melphalan are also effective. These drugs all have the advantage that they can be given by mouth. Other drugs used include 5-fluorouracil, actinomycin D and vinblastine, but these are not as effective as chlorambucil. Combination chemotherapy has not so far shown any definite advantage over single agents in the treatment of this tumour, but clinical trials are in progress and the recently introduced cis-diaminedichloroplatinum has shown promising activity. The results of treatment of ovarian carcinoma vary from a 5-year survival of 60–75 per cent in patients with early disease confined to the ovaries at the time of diagnosis to 0–10 per cent in patients with more widespread disease.

BODY OF THE UTERUS (ENDOMETRIUM)

Carcinoma

This tumour is less common than carcinoma of the cervix and has a later age of onset. The majority of women are post-menopausal and it is uncommon before the age of 45. It is seen more often in nulliparous women and there is an association with diabetes, obesity and hypertension. It is also more common in higher social groups. There is some evidence to suggest a causal relationship with previous oestrogen administration, but this is not yet conclusive.

Pathology

Carcinoma of the body of the uterus arises from the columnar epithelium of the endometrium. It tends to grow and spread slowly, the mass of muscle in the body of the uterus containing its spread. Most tumours are well differentiated and lymphatic involvement (of the pelvic and para-aortic glands) occurs relatively late. Metastases to the lungs, bones, liver and brain occur but are a late feature.

Clinical features

Post-menopausal bleeding is the most important symptom, but menorrhagia or inter-menstrual bleeding before the menopause or the presence of a watery discharge should arouse suspicion. Pain is rare but may occur when there is obstruction to the cervical canal with formation of a pyometrium. Vaginal examination is usually normal with small tumours while enlargement and fixation of the uterus are signs of advanced disease.

Investigations

The diagnosis is established by histological examination of the endo-metrium after curettage. Cytological examination is less useful than with carcinoma of the cervix because exfoliated cells may undergo autolysis in the uterine cavity. Clinical examination and curettage usually indicate the stage of the disease but a chest X-ray is necessary and intravenous urography should be performed if there is any suspicion of spread beyond the uterus.

Treatment

The conventional treatment of a carcinoma of the body of the uterus is total hysterectomy with bilateral salpingo-oophorectomy and in early cases this produces a 5-year survival rate of over 80 per cent. Even with later cases a survival rate of between 60 and 70 per cent may be obtained and the use of radiotherapy either before or after surgery can improve this figure and reduce the incidence of recurrences in the vagina. The prognosis is worsened by the presence of invasion of the myometrium, if the tumour is poorly differentiated or spread to the endocervix or pelvic lymph nodes has occurred. With late disease, much can be achieved by either preliminary radiotherapy followed by a simple hysterectomy or, if this is not feasible, radiation alone. Even when the disease is very advanced locally or when there are pulmonary or bone metastases, remissions lasting several years can sometimes be obtained by using high doses of a progestogen such as medroxyprogesterone 600 mg daily.

Sarcoma

Sarcomas of the uterus are rare but arise either from endometrial stroma cells which infiltrate the myometrium or as a result of malignant change in fibromyomas to produce a leiomyosarcoma. These have generally a poor prognosis except when tumours are well-differentiated, or if, in the case of the endometrial stromal sarcoma, there is some hormone dependence when there may be a response to endocrine therapy after hysterectomy and oophorectomy. The prognosis is better for leiomyosarcoma occurring in younger patients. Treatment consists of total hysterectomy with removal of all visible tumour.

CERVIX UTERI

Carcinoma

This is the commonest tumour of the female genital tract, being second only to carcinoma of the breast as a cause of cancer in women. It is about twice as common as carcinoma of the body of the uterus. It occurs more often in women of low income groups with poor living conditions and bad personal hygiene. Early age of regular intercourse, promiscuity and genital herpes are factors associated with an increased risk of this disease, whereas it is uncommon in virgins and ethnic groups in which men are circumcised. The incidence is low in Israel and Moslem countries and high in parts of South America. There is increasing evidence that a virus infection plays an important part in the aetiology of this tumour and, if this is confirmed, then prevention may be improved in addition to the contribution already made by early detection (screening—see below).

Pathology

Squamous carcinomas account for 95 per cent and arise most often in the squamo-columnar junction. The remainder are adenocarcinomas which arise in the mucus-secreting glands. The tumour may be a nodule or an ulcer which either projects into the cervical canal or infiltrates deeply into the wall of the cervix. The degree of differentiation, from well-keratinised and differentiated cells to small poorly differentiated cells with little keratin, has an important bearing upon the behaviour of the tumour.

Infiltration tends to be lateral, involvement of the bladder anteriorly or the rectum posteriorly being relatively late. With growth into parametrial tissues, obstruction to the ureters is likely. Lymphatic spread occurs to the pelvic, iliac and para-aortic nodes. Blood-borne spread producing metastases in the lung or brain is uncommon, bone metastases being rare.

The staging of carcinoma of the cervix is complicated by discrepancies between the TNM classification and that of the cancer committee of the International Federation of Gynaecology and Obstetrics. The latter, which is used more widely, is as follows:

Stage I.S or O	Carcinoma *in situ*;
Stage Ia	Histological diagnosis only: pre-clinical invasive carcinoma;
Stage Ib	Clinical invasive carcinoma confined to the cervix;
Stage IIa	Spread to the vagina but not the lower third;
Stage IIb	Involvement of the parametrium but not pelvic wall. Vagina can be involved but not the lower third;
Stage IIIa	Involvement of the lower third of the vagina;
Stage IIIb	Involvement of the pelvic wall;
Stage IV	Involvement of the bladder or rectal mucosa or distant metastases.

Detection of pre-clinical cancer by screening

There is little doubt that carcinoma *in situ* (in which the cervix looks normal) may proceed to invasive cancer. However, there is evidence that in some instances spontaneous regression occurs. The diagnosis can be made on the basis of a Papanicolaou smear of exfoliated cervical cells obtained at a screening examination. This procedure has become an important method of enabling early detection, thereby reducing the morbidity and mortality of this disease. Regular cytological examination is recommended for all sexually active women of whatever age, but the optimal intervals between examination are not yet determined. In North America 6- or 12-monthly routine cytological tests are recommended, but in Europe the intervals tend to be longer. The incidence of the various stages at diagnosis varies in different parts of the world, and depends partly upon the screening practices. For instance, in North America approximately 80 per cent of cases are now diagnosed in pre-invasive or early invasive stages, while the incidence of advanced disease is declining. In Europe, however, many cases of Stage III and IV disease are still seen but an increasing awareness of the condition has led to earlier referral, and the wider adoption of cervical cytology should lead to diminishing incidence of advanced disease as now seen in North America.

Clinical features of invasive cancer

The main symptom of carcinoma of the cervix is abnormal bleeding which may be post-coital, inter-menstrual or post-menopausal. A vaginal discharge may be present which can be clear, blood-stained or offensive. Pain is a late feature and suggests involvement of extra-uterine pelvic structures. Other late features are rectal or bladder fistulae, swelling of the legs due to lymphatic obstruction and ureteric obstruction leading to renal failure.

Investigations

Clinical staging is determined by clinical examination. Diagnosis is confirmed by curettage of the uterus and biopsy of the cervix which is essential to confirm the diagnosis. It may also be necessary to undertake cystoscopy. Intravenous urography is performed in all cases together with radiological examination of the chest. Other selected investigations which may be useful are a sigmoidoscopy and barium enema to determine whether or not there is rectal involvement and lymphography to assess the state of the lymph nodes.

Treatment

Radiotherapy and surgery are the most effective means of treatment of carcinoma of the cervix but there is disagreement as to the best approach. The results of either treatment are similar in expert hands. The definitive treatment of carcinoma *in situ* consists of a cone biopsy and careful follow-up in women who want further children, but in other women, hysterectomy may be performed with preservation of the ovaries. For Stage Ia and b and IIa radiotherapy alone is preferred in many centres, but in others pre-operative radiation is given followed by radical (Wertheim) hysterectomy with further radiation if pelvic lymph nodes are involved. For Stage IIb and Stage III radiation therapy alone is given and in the case of Stage IV the treatment will depend upon which structures are involved. Palliative surgical procedures may be necessary in the case of fistulae or ureteric obstruction, and radiotherapy is used when indicated.

Chemotherapy has, so far, proved disappointing in the treatment of carcinoma of the cervix, although alkylating agents, methotrexate, mitomycin C, vincristine, bleomycin and adriamycin have all been used with occasional success.

The 5-year survival rate of patients with carcinoma *in situ* treated surgically approaches 100 per cent and the results are almost the same for Stage Ia. The survival at 5 years for patients with Stages IIb and III disease falls to 30–40 per cent. Even in patients with Stage IV disease the outlook is not always hopeless since with supervoltage radiotherapy a number survive for several years.

Other tumours of the cervix and vagina

Between 5 and 10 per cent of tumours of the cervix are adenocarcinomas which do not have any particular association with the factors known to be concerned with squamous carcinoma. There is, however, one variety, namely the clear-cell adenocarcinoma of the cervix, which is encountered in adolescent girls whose mothers received oestrogen therapy in the early weeks of pregnancy. This is similar to the adenocarcinoma of the vagina which is found in the same circumstances. Adenocarcinomas of the cervix tend to spread more rapidly in the lymphatic system and distant metastases are more common. The treatment is similar to that for squamous carcinoma of the cervix but the results are worse. Occasionally a mixed carcinoma of the cervix is encountered, comprising a combination of squamous and adenocarcinoma. Sarcoma of the cervix is extremely rare and has the worst prognosis of tumours at this site.

VULVA

Tumours of the vulva account for less than 5 per cent of genital cancers and occur predominantly in older women. About 95 per cent are squamous carcinomas but other conditions such as Bowen's disease, Paget's disease, malignant melanoma and adenocarcinoma of the sweat and Bartholin's glands are occasionally encountered. The squamous carcinoma appears as an ulcer or nodule which spreads to surrounding tissues involving the urethra, rectum and bone and by lymphatic spread to the inguinal, femoral and external iliac nodes. The clinical features consist of irritation, pain, discharge and bleeding with ulceration. Biopsy of suspicious lesions is essential to establish the diagnosis and to distinguish it from a variety of benign lesions of the vulva which can give rise to similar symptoms.

Treatment consists of radical vulvectomy with excision of bilateral regional lymph nodes. This operation has a high cure rate and should be undertaken even in old patients as there is a low operative mortality. Small lesions (less than 3 cm diameter) have a 60–80 per cent 5-year survival rate.

CHORIOCARCINOMA

Choriocarcinoma is of great interest since it was the first tumour to be cured by chemotherapy alone. It follows the occurrence of a hydatidiform mole, invasive mole or an apparently normal pregnancy or abortion. The incidence of choriocarcinoma is about 3 per cent following hydatidiform and invasive moles. The incidence after non-molar pregnancy is about one in 50000 amongst Europeans. There is a greater incidence in oriental populations where moles occur more commonly.

Pathology

It is part of the function of the trophoblast to invade the decidua, and trophoblast from a mole may invade as far as the uterine muscle or beyond. Tissue from a mole may be found in the vagina but the main risk of invasion is perforation of the uterus with massive intraperitoneal bleeding. In the case of choriocarcinoma, metastatic spread may be early and widespread with secondary deposits being found in the lungs, brain, gastro-intestinal tract, liver and elsewhere.

Clinical features

The presence of a choriocarcinoma following a mole is recognised by high titres of chorionic gonadotrophin in the urine. In the case of choriocarcinoma following a normal pregnancy the symptoms may be variable and depend on the site of metastases. Pulmonary metastases are present in about 70 per cent of patients and are numerous. It is unusual for breathlessness to be evident but haemoptysis is common. Cerebral metastases may present with features of raised intracranial pressure or an intracerebral haemorrhage. Anaemia may be present due to gastro-intestinal bleeding from metastases.

Investigations

The most important investigation is the measurement of human chorionic gonadotrophin (hCG) in the urine by radio-immuno-assay, which is more specific when the *beta* subfraction is measured. The presence of a choriocarcinoma is suggested by levels of hCG greater than 40000 i.u./day more than four to six weeks following evacuation of a hydatidiform mole or more than 25000 i.u./day after ten weeks; hCG persisting at any level five to seven months later also indicates the presence of a choriocarcinoma.

A chest radiograph is important and a brain scan may be required, other investigations including full haematological and biochemical screening. Pelvic arteriography can be valuable to identify metastases and provide a base-line upon which to assess response to treatment and to assist in selecting patients for hysterectomy.

Treatment

The treatment of choriocarcinoma is greatly facilitated by monitoring levels of hCG in the blood or urine. This marker is still detectable when as few as one million tumour cells remain. Intermittent chemotherapy can therefore be continued beyond this point with a good chance of achieving eradication of the disease. Should this not be achieved then relapsing disease may be detected at an early stage after treatment has been stopped and it can be started again.

Low-risk patients are those recognised within six months of evacuation of hydatidiform mole or with choriocarcinoma diagnosed within three months of a term pregnancy or abortion. Treatment of this group comprises methotrexate alone, which results in cure of 90 per cent of cases. Patients with extensive metastases are a medium-risk group and require more complex regimens of chemotherapy, using several agents including methotrexate, cyclophosphamide, vincristine and actinomycin D. The high-risk group of patients are those in whom pregnancy has occurred two or more years before the start of treatment and those with larger masses of tumour. Such patients require similar chemotherapy for longer periods.

CHAPTER SIXTEEN

ENDOCRINE GLANDS

Endocrine tumours of the pancreas, bowel and gonads have been discussed elsewhere (Chapters 7, 14, 15); those of the pituitary, thyroid and adrenal glands are described here.

PITUITARY

While metastases in the pituitary gland (particularly from the breast) are relatively common, malignant primary tumours do not occur. Benign tumours expand, causing pressure upon the optic chiasma or surrounding structures and may interfere with metabolism as a result of excessive secretion (for example, acromegaly in eosinophil adenomas and Cushing's syndrome with basophil adenomas) or from deficiency of pituitary hormones. Since these are beyond the scope of this chapter they will not be considered further.

Craniopharyngioma. This tumour, which may be solid or cystic, arises above the sella turcica from developmental remnants of Rathke's pouch. It compresses the optic chiasma causing visual field defects and extends upwards into the hypothalamus. It is usually encountered in childhood when it causes arrested growth and diabetes insipidus. Occasionally it presents in adult life and causes hypopituitarism. An enlarged, shallow sella is seen on lateral skull radiographs with, in about 50 per cent of cases, visible flecks of calcification.

THYROID

Metastases, particularly from cancers of the breast, lung and kidney tumours, occur in the thyroid gland, but there are four important types of primary thyroid cancer. These are rare tumours accounting for under 1 per cent of all cancer deaths, being twice as common in women than men. The number of deaths from thyroid cancer in the United Kingdom is about 400 each year.

Pathology

The most common malignant tumour of the thyroid is the *papillary carcinoma* which accounts for approximately 60 per cent of such tumours and is the one found most often in childhood and younger adults. In children it may follow radiotherapy to the neck or nasopharynx, which in some parts of the world has been a common treatment for benign conditions such as adenoid hyperplasia, but usually its cause is not known. The tumour consists of well-differentiated columnar cells forming a solitary nodule in the thyroid gland which spreads to the cervical lymph nodes.

Follicular carcinoma is the next most common form and accounts for approximately 25 per cent. It is well-differentiated and closely resembles normal thyroid tissue, but microscopic examination reveals invasion of blood vessels, the capsule and lymphatics. It occurs more commonly in older patients than papillary carcinoma and metastasises more widely, particularly to bones, brain and lungs.

Anaplastic carcinoma accounts for approximately 10 per cent of thyroid tumours and consists of either squamous cells, spindle cells or small round cells. It occurs predominantly in the elderly, grows rapidly and has a poor prognosis.

Medullary carcinoma is a solid differentiated tumour well-demarcated from the remainder of the thyroid gland, and it arises from the calcitonin-producing 'C' cells. It accounts for about 5 per cent of thyroid tumours and is found in a relatively younger age group with a preponderance of females. This remarkable tumour is associated with several other abnormalities, including neuromas of the tongue, lip and eyelids, and phaeochromocytomas which are often bilateral and familial.

A fifth tumour which is very rare and accounts for only 1 per cent of thyroid neoplasms is a malignant lymphoma.

Clinical features

Thyroid tumours present as swellings of the thyroid gland itself or as metastases. In the case of papillary carcinoma, lymph nodes may be palpable in the neck with a small, clinically undetectable tumour in the gland itself. By contrast, the anaplastic carcinoma grows rapidly and may lead to respiratory obstruction with stridor, requiring emergency surgical relief.

Investigations

A radioisotope (^{125}I or ^{131}I) scan of the gland usually shows a 'cold' nodule since the surrounding normal gland takes up iodine more avidly that the tumour. Radiographs of the chest and bones are necessary to identify the presence of metastases. With medullary carcinomas calcitonin levels are raised excessively in response to an intravenous infusion of calcium; urinary catechol amines will be elevated with co-existing phaeochromocytomas. Needle biopsy has been used to confirm the diagnosis but surgical exploration is safer.

Treatment

The preferred primary treatment is surgical excision with removal of as much of the tumour as possible. In the case of the well-differentiated tumours, which are functionally similar to normal thyroid tissue, remaining tumour either in the gland, lymph nodes or elsewhere can be destroyed by large doses of radioactive iodine. Both papillary and follicular carcinomas are to some extent dependent on thyroid-stimulating hormone and regress when this is suppressed by administering thyroxine.

Anaplastic tumours do not respond to radioactive iodine or thyroxine since they are not functionally active. Surgery is seldom useful except to produce an airway and to establish the diagnosis. Radiotherapy may give useful short remissions but relapse is usually early and the prognosis is poor. Medullary carcinoma is treated by surgical excision of the tumour.

ADRENAL GLANDS

Tumours of the adrenal glands are rare and arise either in the cortex, when they may produce various metabolic effects according to the hormones which are elaborated, or in the medulla as the exceedingly rare malignant phaeochromocytoma.

Carcinoma of the adrenal cortex

Pathology

These tumours, which are initially encapsulated, may become very large and eventually invade the adrenal vein, inferior vena cava and lymphatics. The degree of differentiation is variable, as is their capacity to produce hormones. They account for about 10 per cent of cases of Cushing's syndrome, which is the commonest metabolic consequence of these tumours owing to the excessive production of cortisol. Less often androgens are produced, which cause virilising effects in females and, extremely rarely, oestrogens are produced which cause feminisation in males. They are usually unilateral and functional autonomously so that the contra-lateral gland atrophies due to suppression of adrenocorticotrophin (ACTH) secretion.

Clinical features

The most common features in functioning tumours are those of Cushing's syndrome with truncal obesity, mooning of the face, hypertension and diabetes. Less commonly, when virilisation is the most conspicuous feature, symptoms can be marked and rapidly progressive as, although the adrenal androgens are relatively weak, they are produced in large quantities. Gynaecomastia in males due to a feminising adrenocortical carcinoma is rare. When the tumour is not functioning it is likely to present as a mass in the adrenal region causing local pain and, by involving the kidney, haematuria and infection may occur. Weight loss, anorexia, and fever are often present, and metastases in the skeleton when present usually give rise to pain.

Investigations

Establishing the diagnosis consists of biochemical investigation in those patients with functioning tumours and, in all patients, it is necessary to locate precisely the anatomical site of the tumour. Confirmation of the diagnosis of Cushing's syndrome is made by finding elevated plasma cortisol levels with absent diurnal variation and, in the case of an autonomous tumour, ACTH levels are either low or absent in the plasma. Failure to suppress the raised level of cortisol is seen on administering dexamethasone, and urinary levels of 17-hydroxycorticoids and 17-ketosteroids are very high. The metyrapone test helps to distinguish between hyperplasia and tumours of the adrenal cortex. A variety of radiological investigations have been used successfully to demonstrate the presence of an adrenal tumour. Intravenous urography or peri-renal insufflation of oxygen and carbon dioxide combined with tomography may be used, but selective angiography is now the preferred procedure. More recently scintiscanning has proved useful but it is not widely available. The method consists of using ^{131}I-labelled cholesterol, which is incorporated into the steroids synthesized by the tumour but is not taken up by contralateral adrenal which has suppressed function.

In order to detect the presence of metastases, it is necessary to undertake other investigations such as chest radiographs and bone and liver scans.

Treatment

The adrenal tumour should be explored surgically and resected if possible. It is important to cover the operative and post-operative periods with additional cortisol and fludrocortisone since the remaining adrenal will not be fully functional for some time. Radiotherapy is of some value to relieve pain due to metastases in bone. Metastases elsewhere can be treated with mitotane (O,P'-DDD) which has a cytotoxic action upon the cells of the adrenal cortex. Aminoglutethamide is another drug which is sometimes useful, since it suppresses the metabolic effects of the tumour, although it has no effect upon its growth. Surgical removal of functioning tumours usually results in regression of the clinical features, but recurrence is common. As carcinomas of the adrenal are so uncommon there are few series reported upon which to base survival figures, but on the whole these tumours have a poor prognosis.

Phaeochromocytoma

Malignant phaeochromocytomas are exceedingly rare, accounting for about 10 per cent of all phaeochromocytomas. They arise in the argentaffin cells of the sympathetic nervous system and secrete the hormones adrenaline and noradrenaline. The clinical features are those of hypertension, which may be paroxysmal or sustained and accompanied by palpitations, sweating, blanching of the skin, faintness and headaches. Urinary catechol amines are elevated but the diagnosis is established by aortography with selective injection of adrenal vessels or adrenal vein catheterisation. Treatment consists of surgical removal of the tumour and precautions have to be taken during surgery to control the blood pressure with phenoxybenzamine and adrenergic beta–blockers (e.g. propranolol).

CHAPTER SEVENTEEN

NERVOUS SYSTEM

This chapter concerns tumours affecting the brain, spinal cord, peripheral nerves and eye. The closely related diseases, meningeal leukaemia, pituitary gland tumours and neuroblastoma, are considered elsewhere (Chapters 9, 16 and 19 respectively). In addition, non-metastatic neurological manifestations of cancer are described.

BRAIN

The incidence of malignant brain tumours with respect to age shows two peaks, one in childhood, when tumours occur predominantly infratentorially, and a second peak in middle age when the majority are situated above the tentorium. Because of the rigidity of the skull and the injurious effect of compression on brain tissue, brain tumours may cause severe neurological dysfunction and be fatal when only of modest size in comparison with tumours occurring elsewhere.

Pathology

Only two intracranial neoplasms can be considered to be benign in that they are encapsulated and, usually, amenable to complete surgical excision; they are not, moreover, true brain tumours. These are meningioma and acoustic neuroma. The majority of primary brain tumours arise from the glial-supporting cells of the brain and are known collectively as gliomas. Although it is exceedingly rare for primary brain tumours to metastasise distantly, the majority are considered malignant because they are locally invasive.

Meningioma. Meningiomas occur principally in middle age and account for a small minority of intracranial tumours. They arise in the meninges, where they can occur at any site, but are most commonly situated parasaggittally, along the sphenoidal ridge, in the olfactory groove and in the parasellar region. When situated in the vault of the cranium, hypertrophic periosteal changes frequently occur in the overlying skull. Usually benign, these tumours occasionally undergo sarcomatous change and assume the characteristics of malignancy.

Neurilemmoma (schwannoma, acoustic neuroma). Acoustic neuromas occur about three times more frequently in females than in males and account for about 6 per cent of intracranial tumours. They are sometimes bilateral, and may occur in association with neurofibromatosis. They arise in the sheath of the eighth cranial nerve and cause a variety of syndromes including unilateral deafness, tinnitus, vertigo, headache and hydrocephalus. Characteristic widening of the internal auditory meatus in the petrous bone can be identified in the appropriate radiographs.

Glioma. Gliomas account for about 40 per cent of primary brain tumours. Histologically, they show a broad spectrum of differentiation and, since they are not encapsulated, the margins of these tumours are frequently difficult to determine. Various distinct types of glioma are described.

Malignant astrocytoma (glioblastoma multiforme).   This is the most common glioma and is usually highly malignant, causing early death (10 per cent survival at 18 months from diagnosis). Other types of astrocytoma occur with lower degrees of malignancy and proportionately longer survival.

Ependymoma.   These uncommon tumours, accounting for about 4 per cent of all gliomas, arise from the epithelial lining of the ventricles and occur usually in children and young adults, when the most common site is in the fourth ventricle. Ependymomas are the commonest gliomas of the spinal cord. The prognosis of patients with ependymomas is largely dependent on the site of the tumour and suitability for surgical excision. When this is favourable the median survival is as high as 10 years.

Oligodendroglioma.   These gliomas are also uncommon and occur principally in middle life when they are situated predominantly in the cerebral hemispheres. They are slowly growing tumours, often demonstrating calcification, and have a good prognosis with a median survival of 4 or 5 years, but some patients may survive as long as 20 years.

Medulloblastoma.   This is the commonest brain tumour occurring in children. The majority of medulloblastomas are situated infratentorially, the cerebellum and fourth ventricle being usually involved. Medulloblastomas metastasise to other parts of the central nervous system through the cerebrospinal fluid. These tumours are usually responsive to treatment and the median survival is about five years.

Metastases in the brain. Primary tumours outside the nervous system commonly metastasise to the brain; for example, over half of patients dying of malignant melanoma are found to have cerebral metastases at autopsy. Other tumours frequently metastasising to the brain are carcinomas of the lung, breast, kidney, head and neck, and thyroid.

Clinical features

The clinical features of intracranial neoplasms depend upon their site and the rapidity of growth. Typically the history is of progressive disturbance of neurological function over a period of months or weeks but occasionally it is much shorter. The brain and its membranes are enclosed within the rigid skull so that the increasing size of a tumour is eventually likely to lead to a rise in intracranial pressure. This produces headaches and vomiting and often, but not always, papilloedema, which are liable to occur early with growths in the posterior cranial fossa because of obstruction to the normal flow of cerebro-spinal fluid.

Mental symptoms may follow the rise in intracranial pressure with apathy and intellectual impairment progressing eventually to drowsiness and finally coma. Tumours involving the cerebral hemispheres may cause epilepsy and the pattern of seizures with sensorimotor or complex visual or olfactory symptoms sometimes permits an accurate prediction of the site of the lesion. Parietal lobe involvement causes contralateral hemianaesthesia or sensory inattention with aphasia, agnosia and apraxia if the dominant hemisphere is involved. Frontal lobe tumours may be 'silent' but tend to produce a progressive dementia unless the motor cortex or Broca's area are involved resulting in Jacksonian seizures, hemiparesis or aphasia.

Investigations

Although the clinical features of brain tumours can often accurately indicate the site of the tumour, further investigations are required for precise localisation. It must be stressed, however, that these investigations only assist in confirming the nature and site of the disease; the histological diagnosis must await biopsy obtained at either burr-hole examination or craniotomy. Lumbar puncture should not be performed when there is evidence of raised intracranial pressure because of the danger of 'coning' and plays virtually no part in the investigation of suspected intracranial tumour.

Skull radiograph. Features seen on plain radiography of the skull which may indicate the presence of an intracranial tumour include widening of the sutures (in children only), erosion of bones of the dorsum sellae with erosion of the posterior clinoid processes, or shift of a visibly calcified pineal gland from the midline. Calcification, sometimes seen in tumours, is usually an indication of slow growth.

Electroencephalogram (EEG). For supratentorial tumours, disturbances in the electroencephalographic pattern may indicate, and help to localise, the site of a tumour. This safe, non-invasive investigation is useful in patients with epileptic seizures to determine whether an abnormal and localised focus is present, but does not indicate the pathological cause of such a focus.

Echo-encephalography. Echo-encephalography with ultrasound is also a safe, non-invasive procedure which may localise intracranial tumours. However, for the best results the investigation needs a high degree of skill, and the technique has not been widely adopted.

Isotopic brain scanning. Because of their vascularity and altered vascular permeability, most brain tumours show increased uptake of radioactive isotope after intravenous injection. The most commonly used isotope is technetium (^{99m}Tc). Brain scanning is likely to give positive results with the more vascular tumours such as malignant astrocytoma, meningioma and cerebral metastases; false negative results may be obtained with more slowly growing avascular tumours and after corticosteroids have been given. Tumours smaller than 2 cm diameter cannot usually be detected with this technique.

Computerised tomography (CT scanning). This relatively new technique has largely replaced the invasive, more risky investigations of angiography and air encephalography (see below).

With this technique a patient's head is scanned by an X-ray beam in multiple planes, sequentially, and the X-ray absorption at numerous positions is calculated by a computer. Horizontal sections of the brain anatomy can then be displayed on a cathode-ray tube and photographed for permanent recording. Brain tumours are seen as areas of increased attenuation compared to normal brain, and the definition of the lesions can be sharpened considerably by repeating the CT scan after the intravenous injection of iodine-containing contrast media. The time required for CT scanning is short compared with arteriography and air encephalography, and is more readily repeated at intervals; the radiation dosage is also lower.

Cerebral angiography. Until the introduction of computerised tomography, cerebral angiography was the most valuable and accurate diagnostic procedure in the investigation of brain tumours. In this technique a radio-opaque contrast medium is injected into the carotid or vertebral arteries, under either local or general anaesthesia, after which serial radiographs are taken. In the presence of a cerebral neoplasm, angiography may show either displacement of the normal vessels, a pathological tumour circulation, or both.

Air encephalography. Air was the first contrast medium to be used in the radiological study of intracerebral neoplasms. In air encephalography, air is injected into the cerebrospinal fluid space through a lumbar-puncture needle, but this technique is hazardous in patients with cerebral tumours who are in danger of 'coning'. In that case, an alternative procedure, ventriculography, in which air was inserted into the ventricles via a burr-hole, used to be employed in neurosurgical units. Both techniques have been largely replaced by computerised tomography. Air encephalography is still necessary for the determination of small, suprasellar tumours.

Treatment

The optimal treatment of cerebral tumours depends upon their histology and location and may involve surgery, radiotherapy and/or chemotherapy. If the patient is in danger of coning, urgent treatment of cerebral oedema is mandatory. Large doses of intravenous corticosteroids, particularly agents which cause little sodium retention such as dexamethasone, are employed. Osmotic diuretics, such as mannitol, may also be used but only under neurosurgical supervision because of the danger of 'rebound' oedema following their withdrawal. Anticonvulsant therapy with phenytoin and/or phenobarbitone may be needed to control epileptic seizures.

Surgery. Although many tumours are not curable by surgery, confirmation of the clinical and radiological diagnosis by craniotomy and biopsy after the appropriate investigations is usually necessary to determine the precise histological diagnosis, and to ensure that a curable condition has not been missed. Curative excision is usually possible for meningiomas and acoustic neuromas, but the operative mortality may be relatively high. For malignant tumours which are not completely resectable, surgery may provide worthwhile palliation. The extent and feasibility of surgery depend largely on the site of the tumour and the functional importance of the surrounding brain tissue. Surgical excision of single, discrete metastases from tumours elsewhere (particularly carcinoma of the bronchus) may sometimes result in relief of symptoms and prolonged survival. The results of surgery are better if pre-operative treatment, particularly for cerebral oedema, has been adequate. Cerebral tumours are often highly vascular and blood transfusion may be required during operation.

Radiotherapy. The place of radiotherapy in treating primary brain tumours is controversial; patients are often selected because surgical treatment is not feasible. There is disagreement regarding the value of radiotherapy after surgical excision and controlled trials are needed to settle this point, but it is useful to provide palliation with inoperable tumours. Medulloblastoma, however, is a highly radiosensitive tumour and, because of the tendency of this tumour to metastasise throughout the central nervous system, resection should be followed by post-operative craniospinal irradiation. Radiotherapy is often the appropriate treatment for cerebral metastases whose responsiveness depends on the history of the primary tumour.

Chemotherapy. Although primary brain tumours remain confined almost invariably to the central nervous system, local treatment (surgery and radiotherapy) alone frequently fails to eradicate them. There is interest, therefore, in the use of chemotherapeutic agents, but little information is available at the present time and controlled trials have only recently begun. Although the majority of cytotoxic drugs are not lipid-soluble, this may be of less importance than was once believed, because the endothelial lining between the blood and brain tumour tissue is much more permeable than the normal 'blood–brain barrier'. However, the lipid-soluble nitrosoureas are of particular interest and recent studies have shown that they can cause regression of some of these tumours. Methotrexate, administered intrathecally, is of proven value in the treatment of medulloblastoma and some tumours which metastasise to the central nervous system, particularly acute lymphoblastic leukaemia. Vincristine appears to be of some value, but information available concerning other agents (cyclophosphamide, 5-fluorouracil, mustine) is not encouraging.

SPINAL CORD

Tumours involving the spinal cord are classified as either extradural or intradural. Extradural tumours include metastases from solid tumours, myeloma, lymphomas and miscellaneous sarcomas. The intradural tumours are subdivided further into the extramedullary tumours (neurofibroma, meningioma) and intramedullary (glioma, particularly ependymoma, and haemangioma). The majority of tumours involving the spinal cord are extradural, being metastases from primary tumours elsewhere, particularly the bronchus, breast, prostate, kidney and gastro-intestinal tract. Primary tumours of the spinal cord are rare.

Because there is little space for spinal-cord displacement, small tumours may result in severe disturbance of neurological function. Pain is a common presenting symptom and may be particularly well-localised if dorsal roots are involved, but tumours placed centrally within the cord produce more diffuse pain. Typically, tumours affecting the spinal cord cause motor and sensory loss at, and below, the neurological segment of involvement. Lateral spinal-cord compression may cause a Brown–Sequard syndrome (ipsilateral motor loss and spasticity together with loss of light touch, vibration and position sense, associated with contralateral loss of pain and temperature sensation). As spinal-cord lesions progress, spasticity and weakness become bilateral and bowel and urinary bladder dysfunction occur. It is essential for spinal-cord compression to be recognised as an acute emergency, as it may be reversed by treatment if detected early in its development. A few hours delay may adversely affect the prognosis because recovery of spinal-cord function is improbable once motor loss and sphincter disturbance have become established. As soon as spinal-cord compression is suspected, patients should be transferred to a neurosurgical unit for myelography with the utmost urgency and if the diagnosis is confirmed, a laminectomy is performed at the appropriate level in order to decompress the cord and remove as much tumour as possible. Post-operatively it is expedient to irradiate the site of involvement. This situation is no less urgent if a patient is known to have metastatic carcinoma since paraplegia can only add to the distress of the illness and can usually be avoided by prompt treatment.

PERIPHERAL NERVES

Primary tumours of peripheral nerves are rare. They are usually benign and arise from the Schwann cells of the nerve sheaths (schwannoma; neurilemmoma); only rarely do they become malignant. Similar neoplasms, the neurofibromas, also usually benign and occurring as single lesions, are occasionally multiple in association with von Recklinghausen's neurofibromatosis. Sarcomatous change in a neurofibroma is a rare event, but fibrosarcomas may develop in the peripheral nerves. Malignant tumours of neural crest remnants in ganglia (neuroblastoma) occur in childhood (Chapter 19).

EYE

The eye and its surroundings are not commonly involved in malignant disease but a large variety of neoplasms may occur in this region. The investigation and management of these conditions is highly specialised and only a brief summary is given.

Eyelids

The most common tumour to involve the eyelids are basal-cell carcinomas; less commonly, squamous-cell carcinoma and malignant melanoma occur. Treatment of these conditions is usually by surgical excision, radiotherapy or both. Biopsy should always be done before radical treatment is undertaken as these lesions may clinically resemble kerato-acanthoma, which usually regresses spontaneously.

Orbit

Many neoplastic, and non-neoplastic, conditions arise in the orbit which are characterised by proptosis and extra-ocular muscle dysfunction. By far the most common malignant tumours are lymphomas in adults, and embryonal rhabdomyosarcoma in children. Gliomas and neurilemmomas occur in the optic nerve but are uncommon. Carcinomas may arise in the lacrimal gland.

Investigation of value in the diagnosis of orbital lesions are skull radiograph, tomography, orbital phlebography and computerised tomography; histological examination of a biopsy specimen is essential. The correct treatment of lesions in the orbit depends on their nature and extent. Some tumours may be curable by radiotherapy, particularly malignant lymphomas and embryonal rhabdomyosarcoma, but surgery is often required.

Eyeball

Although rare, the most common tumours to arise primarily in the eyeball are retinoblastoma and malignant melanoma.

Retinoblastoma

This primary tumour of the retina occurs in early life, the mean age at diagnosis being 17 months. It is transmitted genetically as an autosomal dominant, most cases being sporadic mutations with a high degree of gene penetrance. Retinoblastoma may affect one or both eyes; in 80 per cent of cases it is multicentric.

The usual presenting sign of this disease is a white appearance in the pupil and there is often co-existing strabismus. Less commonly the eye may be red and painful, sometimes with the presence of glaucoma or orbital cellulitis. The diagnosis is usually confirmed by ophthalmoscopic examination under anaesthetic. These tumours often contain calcium and aggregates of detached cells may be seen floating in the vitreous, giving rise to seeding elsewhere in the retina. Retinal detachment may occur. The affected eye is often permanently destroyed and the treatment is enucleation. However, because of the tendency of the disease to affect both eyes, the contralateral, ostensibly unaffected, eye should also be treated by radiotherapy as part of the primary treatment. Subsequent recurrences in the retina may be treated by light coagulation, cryotherapy or further radiotherapy. When the disease is diagnosed early, and confined to the eye, the cure rate is as high as 90 per cent or more.

Rarely, retinoblastoma may extend outside the eye along the optic nerve to the brain and meninges and disseminate through the blood forming metastases elsewhere in the body. In these circumstances useful palliation may be achieved with cytotoxic drugs, such as cyclophosphamide and vincristine, or by radiotherapy to certain areas, particularly bony metastases.

Malignant melanoma

Malignant melanoma is the most common primary intra-ocular tumour in adults. Often these tumours are disseminated at the time of diagnosis, particularly if the primary tumour arises in either the choroid or ciliary body, the 5-year survival being about 50 per cent. Tumours arising in the iris grow more slowly, have a better prognosis and can be treated by conservative surgery.

Choroidal melanomas are more difficult to diagnose as they may be confused with retinal haematomas, choroidal haemangiomas or metastatic tumours (particularly from carcinoma of the breast in women, or bronchus in men). These tumours may lead to retinal detachment and visual disturbances, and ophthalmoscopically there is characteristically an elevated lesion with variable amounts of pigmentation. Ultrasonography and isotopic scanning are sometimes useful in the diagnosis of these lesions.

Although enucleation of the eye is often the proper treatment, it may be postponed if vision in the affected eye is good and that of the unaffected eye is impaired. Radiation therapy and light coagulation are also helpful in the treatment of this disease.

NON-METASTATIC NEUROLOGICAL MANIFESTATIONS OF CANCER

Several neurological conditions develop in patients with malignant disease which are not related to metastases in the brain or spinal cord and can precede evidence of the primary growth by long periods, occasionally years. The cause of these disorders is unknown, but has been ascribed to a variety of possible factors including nutritional deficiency, metabolic disturbances, infection of the nervous system by slow viruses and abnormal immune responses. Bronchial carcinoma is the tumour most often found in association with these neurological manifestations but cancers of the ovary, breast, stomach, bowel and uterus may be responsible.

Neuropathy and myopathy. A subacute sensory or sensory and motor neuropathy are not uncommon. Very occasionally spontaneous remission occurs but more usually it progresses. Distal parasthesiae, often painful, and numbness affecting the feet and then the hands are the common presenting symptoms. The development of such a sensory neuropathy in a middle-aged or elderly patient should lead to the suspicion of a carcinoma. Distal wasting and weakness due to simultaneous involvement of motor fibres may also occur.

Asymptomatic proximal wasting and weakness with loss of ankle reflexes and minor sensory impairment are sometimes discovered on routine examination of patients with carcinoma. These cases are commonly called 'carcinomatous neuromyopathy' since both nerve and muscle are thought to be involved, but this is a poorly defined disorder.

The occurrence of progressive proximal wasting and weakness due to inflammation of the muscles, polymyositis, is frequently associated with carcinoma, particularly in the elderly. The muscles are often, but not always painful and tender, the creatine phosphokinase is usually raised and electromyography shows a myopathic pattern. In some cases a character-istic mauve discoloration of the skin of the knuckles and the periorbital region assists the diagnosis and this association is called dermatomyositis. Treatment of carcinomatous myositis with steroids may be beneficial, but is not as satisfactory as the treatment of polymyositis in the absence of carcinoma.

On rare occasions fatigue and weakness associated with carcinoma are due to a neuromuscular block (Eaton–Lambert syndrome) which, unlike myasthenia gravis, is not usually helped by anticholinergic drugs. The reflexes are reduced or absent at rest but are increased after exertion of the muscles. There are specific electromyographic features in this condition and the patient may be improved by treatment with guanidine 20 mg/kg daily.

There may be marked wasting of muscle in the cachexia of advanced malignant disease but power is retained surprisingly well in these circum-stances until relatively late. Muscle weakness may also occur due to hyponatraemia or Cushing's syndrome (Chapter 21).

Other manifestations. Rarely a rapidly progressive cerebellar syndrome or dementia or a combination of both are encountered with carcinoma. Pathologically these are associated with a combination of degeneration and inflammation and the investigation which is most useful to distinguish such lesions from metastases is computerised tomography.

Another very rare syndrome, acute necrotic myelopathy, produces a rapidly progressive tetra- or paraparesis with sensory loss and sphincter involvement. This can only be distinguished from cord compression by myelography.

Progressive multifocal leukoencephalopathy is characterised by multiple foci of demyelination in the brain, cerebellum and brain stem which tend to coalesce. The typical manifestations depend upon the sites of the lesion and are varied. The syndrome is most often found in patients with lymphoma, especially Hodgkin's disease: impaired immunity permits the growth of a polyoma virus in the oligodendrocytes and leads to demyelination. The demyelinated foci can be demonstrated by computerised tomography. Reports of successful treatment with cytosine arabinoside have appeared.

CHAPTER EIGHTEEN

MESENCHYMAL TISSUES

The cells of the embryonal mesenchyme differentiate to form many tissues including the so-called soft tissues (fibrous and adipose tissue, blood and lymph vessels, synovium, smooth and striated muscles), cartilage and bone. Although, collectively, these tissues form well over half the body weight, malignant tumours arising within them are relatively rare. Most of these cancers are designated **sarcomas.**

SOFT TISSUES

Excluding leukaemias and lymphomas, which are considered elsewhere (Chapters 9 and 10), soft-tissue sarcomas account for less than 1 per cent of all cancers, being relatively more frequent in the young than the common carcinomas of older age groups.

The cause of these sarcomas is obscure, although recent immunological and morphological investigations have suggested in some the possibility of a viral aetiology.

Pathology

Malignant tumours arising in soft tissues are much less common than benign growths.

Pathologically the sarcomas are classified according to the tissue of origin and the nomenclature is shown in Table 18.1. The pathologist often needs considerable expertise to identify accurately these tumours, and they are often too anaplastic to permit precise histological classification.

Soft-tissue sarcomas may develop anywhere in the body, and, unlike their benign counterparts, they are not encapsulated, although a pseudo-capsule may be formed around them from compressed tissue. Locally, these tumours invade surrounding structures or extend along nerve sheaths or fascial planes, a factor which makes local recurrence, following limited excision, a common feature. Metastasis to regional lymph nodes and through the blood stream, particularly to the lungs, is common.

The most common soft-tissue sarcomas are liposarcomas and fibrosarcomas. **Liposarcomas**, which frequently have a pseudo-capsule, may grow to very large size and are particularly common in the thigh. There is an increasing incidence of this tumour with age. Liposarcomas differ from benign lipomas in that they are firmer, more deeply situated and less mobile. The prognosis depends largely on the differentiation of the tumour; the 5-year survival for differentiated liposarcomas is about 80 per cent but for anaplastic lesions this falls to 20 per cent. **Fibrosarcomas** may arise at any site and their prognosis is similarly related to the degree of differentiation.

The **rhabdomyosarcomas** form a group of tumours which comprise the third most common soft-tissue sarcoma. Four histological types of rhabdomyosarcoma are generally considered. The *pleomorphic*, which is the most common, usually occurs after the age of 30 and is especially common in males. This type may have a multicentric origin within the same muscle. The *aveolar* rhabdomyosarcoma is highly malignant, occurring predominantly in adolsecents and young adults. The *embryonal* rhabdomyosarcoma is seen principally in the head and neck region, especially within the orbit in children under the age of 10 years, while *botryoidal* tumours are also seen in young children when they usually produce polypoid masses within the genito-urinary tract.

TABLE 18.1   Soft-tissue sarcomas

Tissue or origin	Malignant tumour
Adipose tissue	Liposarcoma
Fibrous tissue	Fibrosarcoma
Striated muscle	Rhabdomyosarcoma
Smooth muscle	Leiomyosarcoma
Synovium	Malignant synovioma (synovial sarcoma)
Undifferentiated mesenchyme	Myxosarcoma
Blood vessels	Angiosarcoma
	Haemangiopericytoma
Lymph vessels	Lymphangiosarcoma
	Kaposi's sarcoma

The other soft-tissue sarcomas are very rare. Malignant synoviomas tend to be situated in the hands, feet or knees; they show a marked tendency to recur locally after excision, and disseminate widely. Myxosarcomas, which arise from undifferentiated mesenchyme, enlarge and infiltrate locally and may reach large size, but unlike the other sarcomas, they do not metastasise distantly. Haemangiopericytomas are typically situated in the nail beds, but this tumour, when sited in the renal glomeruli, has been observed in association with excessive renin production and consequent hypertension. Lymphangiosarcomas have been described as developing in oedematous upper limbs after radical mastectomy for carcinoma of the breast, but this is exceedingly rare. Kaposi's sarcoma, also arising in association with lymph vessels, is seen particularly in certain areas of Africa and is predominantly cutaneous in distribution, although visceral disease also occurs.

Clinical features and diagnosis

Clinically, the soft-tissue sarcomas have the common feature of presenting as progressively enlarging, usually painless, masses. Their rate of growth is variable and because of their frequent deceptively innocent initial appearance and relative rarity, the diagnosis is often delayed for six to twelve months from the onset of symptoms. The diagnosis depends upon the histological examination of a biopsy specimen, particularly to distinguish the malignant nature of the tumour from the more common benign forms. Radiographic studies may also be of value in delineating the extent of soft-tissue sarcomas, and a plain chest radiograph to detect pulmonary metastases is of particular value.

Treatment

Because of the rarity of soft-tissue sarcomas, there is little information concerning treatment which has been derived from controlled clinical trials. However, it is generally accepted that they should be treated by wide surgical excision and occasionally an amputation is required. The radiosensitivity of these tumours is variable, liposarcomas and embryonal rhabdomyosarcomas being particularly radiosensitive, while fibrosarcomas are resistant. Radiotherapy is occasionally selected as the primary treatment for these tumours, after which previously unresectable tumours may become surgically removable, and there is probably an important role for post-operative radiotherapy with primarily operable disease.

Chemotherapy is becoming increasingly useful in the treatment of soft-tissue sarcomas. Methotrexate, as a single agent, has produced short, worth-while remissions in a few patients, but more recently other agents, particularly used in combinations, have shown greater effectiveness. In particular, embryonal rhabdomyosarcoma has proved to be very sensitive to a combination of vincristine, actinomycin D and cyclophosphamide. Adriamycin has also been found of value in a wide variety of sarcomas and is probably more effective in combination with dacarbazine, with a possibility that adding vincristine and cyclophosphamide further increases the response rate. It is probable that further improvements in the treatment of these tumours will be achieved with chemotherapy, especially when used in the primary management in conjunction with local therapy.

BONE AND CARTILAGE

Although the skeleton is commonly involved in malignant disease by metastases from primary tumours elsewhere (particularly carcinomas of the breast, lung, prostate, thyroid), primary cancers of bone account for less than 1 per cent of all malignant tumours (when myelomatosis is excluded). Primary bone cancers are either osseous or non-osseous in origin, the different types being listed in Table 18.2. Osteosarcoma and Ewing's sarcoma are seen predominantly in children, adolescents and young adults under the age of 25, but the other bone tumours have a wide age range. The most useful initial investigation in the diagnosis of bone tumours is plain radiography, but precise diagnosis depends upon histological examination of tissue taken at biopsy.

Osteosarcoma

Osteosarcoma is a cancer developing from bone-forming mesenchyme. The peak incidence is between the ages of 10 and 25 and the disease is most common in males. The most frequent site of involvement is the lower end of the femur and the next most common sites are the tibia and humerus, these areas accounting for 85 per cent of cases. Pathologically, this tumour comprises a sarcomatous stroma in which there is osteoid formation. Predisposing factors include previous exposure to ionising radiation (e.g. after radiotherapy, in watch-dial painters and in persons handling certain radioactive isotopes). In addition a small proportion of patients with Paget's disease of the bone develop osteosarcoma.

Clinically, this tumour is characterised by pain, tenderness and swelling at the site of the tumour, and there is elevation of serum alkaline phosphatase. Radiologically, sclerotic expansion of the bone is usually seen with periosteal extension and, sometimes, a surrounding soft-tissue mass; about 15 per cent of cases illustrate the characteristic 'sun-ray' spiculation appearance.

TABLE 18.2   Primary bone cancer

Osseous	Non-osseous
Osteosarcoma	Fibrosarcoma
Parosteal osteosarcoma	Ewing's sarcoma
Chondrosarcoma	Reticulum-cell sarcoma
Malignant giant-cell tumour	Chordoma
	Angiosarcoma
	Liposarcoma
	Adamantinoma

The usual treatment for this tumour is amputation, but most patients have demonstrable pulmonary metastases within a year of operation, and the 5-year survival after operation is about 20 per cent. The role of radiotherapy in the primary management of this disease has been investigated, particularly pre-operatively, but this has not resulted in improved survival. The advanced disease is occasionally responsive, for brief periods, to a variety of cytotoxic agents including cyclophosphamide, methotrexate, actinomycin D, vincristine and adriamycin. Some recent studies have indicated that post-operative adjuvant chemotherapy, with methotrexate or adriamycin, may improve the prognosis, but confirmatory evidence from controlled studies is not yet available.

Parosteal osteosarcoma

Parosteal osteosarcoma develops on the surface of bones, rather than from the interior of the cortex. Sites of recurrence are similar to those of osteosarcoma, but this is a more slowly growing tumour, often painless, which may reach a large size. It is very radio-opaque. Because of its tendency to recur locally, the preferred treatment is amputation. Although distant metastases may occur, this is uncommon, and the cure rate for this tumour is as high as 80 per cent.

Chondrosarcoma

Chondrosarcoma is a malignant tumour developing in cartilage. It is more common in males and occurs principally in middle age. The sites most affected are the pelvis, proximal femur, ribs and shoulder girdle. Chondrosarcomas grow slowly and are usually painless. Radiologically they are often calcified and poorly defined. They are locally invasive, but distant metastases are uncommon. Cure of these tumours can only be obtained if adequate resection is surgically feasible. These tumours are not radiosensitive and palliative radiotherapy is reserved for inoperable situations. Chemotherapy has been ineffective.

Ewing's sarcoma

This is a highly cellular anaplastic primary sarcoma arising in bone, characterised histologically by a uniform appearance of poorly defined small round cells. Age incidence for this disease is between 10 and 20 years and over 90 per cent of cases occur under the age of 30; the disease is more common in males than in females. The most common bone to be affected is the femur, but any part of the skeleton can give rise to this tumour.

Clinically, Ewing's sarcoma is characterised by pain and a tender swelling at the site of the tumour; fever and weight loss are common. Radiologically there is patchy, lytic bone destruction at the site of the tumour and multiple layering of sub-periosteal new bone formation gives the characteristic 'onion-skin' appearance.

Most patients eventually develop metastases but in about a quarter of cases they are present (usually in the lungs) at the time of diagnosis. Amputation used to be standard treatment, but the 5-year survival rate after surgery alone is less than 10 per cent. Ewing's sarcoma is highly radiosensitive and this is now the preferred local therapy. To effect adequate local control, it is necessary for the whole bone containing the tumour to be irradiated. There is some indication that the whole-body irradiation at lower dosage to eradicate metastatic disease may improve prognosis. Ewing's sarcoma is responsive to a variety of cytotoxic drugs including cyclophosphamide, nitrosoureas, actinomycin D, vincristine and adriamycin, and it is probable that chemotherapy in conjunction with local radiotherapy as primary treatment will improve the prognosis.

Reticulum-cell sarcoma

Histiocytic lymphomas are discussed more fully in Chapter 10, but reticulum-cell sarcoma occasionally arises in, and remains confined to, bone. This tumour may arise at any site in the skeleton, is characterised by relatively slow growth, and ultimately becomes painful with overlying heat and tenderness. In a small proportion of cases, regional lymph nodes are involved and distant metastases in other bones and elsewhere, particularly in the lungs, may be evident. The local tumour can be effectively treated by radiotherapy; chemotherapy, as described for the histiocytic lymphomas, should be given for disseminated disease.

Chordoma

This malignant tumour, arising from remnants of the embryonic notochord, is seen most commonly in late adult life. 80 per cent of these tumours occur in either the occipital or sacro-coccygeal area, the remainder occurring along the vertebral column.

The clinical features depend on the site of the tumour and symptoms may result from nerve-root or spinal-cord compression, while lesions at the base of the spine often cause constipation from rectal compression. Lesions in the occipital area may give rise to disturbance of vision. Radiologically, extensive bone destruction is seen at the site of the tumour.

The preferred treatment for these tumours is usually surgical excision, but when this is not possible, radiotherapy is helpful. After treatment recurrent local disease is common, but distant metastases are rare.

CHAPTER NINETEEN

EMBRYONAL TISSUES

Tumours derived from embryonal tissues are seen principally in young children. The commonest is neuroblastoma followed by nephroblastoma (Wilms' tumour); these and hepatoblastoma are discussed in this chapter. Other embryonal tumours and malignant diseases of children are described elsewhere.

NEUROBLASTOMA

Neuroblastoma is the most common embryonal tumour of childhood. It develops in neural crest cells and so arises in sympathetic ganglia and adrenal medulla, but not the brain or spinal cord. It occurs most often in children under 4 years of age and is exceedingly rare after the age of 14.

Pathology

The cellular differentiation of neuroblastoma varies from a well-differentiated tumour, resembling benign ganglioneuroma, to an anaplastic tumour with no suggestion of neural differentiation. The primary tumour is highly invasive locally and rapidly involves surrounding structures. Regional spread to lymph nodes is common and blood-borne dissemination occurs, most frequently to bone and bone marrow and also to liver; metastases to lungs and brain are rare.

Clinical features

The clinical manifestations of neuroblastoma are protean and depend on the site and extent of the tumour. When neuroblastoma is widespread, there is usually malaise, pallor, weight loss, and sometimes fever. Tumours arising from sympathetic ganglia in the thorax may cause dyspnoea, cough and respiratory infections, while extension of the tumour into the vertebral canal leads to neurological disturbances and, eventually, paraplegia. A tumour developing in the adrenal medulla presents as an abdominal mass which may be confused clinically with Wilms' tumour; liver metastases may simulate hepatoblastoma.

Skeletal metastases cause bone pain and joint swellings, while marrow involvement results in anaemia and bruising from thrombocytopenia. Lymphatic involvement is common, giving rise to mediastinal masses and enlarged supraclavicular nodes.

Investigations

The differential diagnosis of neuroblastoma includes Wilms' tumour and hepatoblastoma; in its disseminated form there may be confusion with acute lymphoblastic leukaemia. However, 90 per cent of patients with neuroblastoma excrete excessive quantities of vanilyl mandelic acid (VMA) in the urine and this provides a useful screening test which, when positive, strongly suggests the diagnosis. Estimation of other catechol amine metabolites may give similar information.

Anaemia, thrombocytopenia and leukopenia may be present as a consequence of widespread bony metastases. Histological confirmation of the disease is very often obtainable on examination of the bone marrow, biopsy of which should be performed in all patients suspected of having neuroblastoma. In addition the skeleton should be surveyed either radiographically or by isotopic scanning. Chest radiography shows the presence of a primary intrathoracic neuroblastoma as a posterior mediastinal mass, usually situated paravertebrally and associated with erosion of ribs and vertebrae. An intravenous urogram is useful to differentiate between neuroblastoma arising in an adrenal gland and a Wilms' tumour, as in the former there is displacement of the kidney downwards, but the calyceal pattern remains normal in contradistinction to Wilms' tumour.

Staging

After clinical examination, investigations and before planning management, the neuroblastoma is staged. A suitable system, which incorporates aspects of other described staging methods, follows:

Stage I   localised tumour which is completely resectable surgically;
Stage II   tumour with regional lymph-node involvement, completely resectable surgically;
Stage III   tumour with regional lymph-node involvement, *not* completely resectable surgically;
Stage IV   distant metastatic disease.
            A—without bone or bone marrow involvement
            B—bone or bone marrow involved

A further stage (IVS) is described, which includes patients who would otherwise be classified as Stage 1 or 2 except that they have distant disease confined to one or more of the following sites only: liver, skin, or bone marrow (without radiographic evidence of bone metastases on complete skeletal survey). Stage IVS disease is particularly common in infants and is associated with a surprisingly good prognosis.

Treatment

The appropriate treatment of neuroblastoma depends on its staging. Because of its aggressive nature Stage I and II disease is uncommon, but surgical excision may be possible for these stages. After complete or partial resection, post-operative radiotherapy is given to the primary site to reduce the chance of local recurrence. The radiotherapy field should be wide enough to include all local disease, and if the vertebral column is in the field, this must be irradiated across its whole width to avoid the development of a scoliosis. Irradiation of kidneys is often unavoidable, but should be reduced to a minimum. Radiotherapy may be used primarily to treat inoperable tumours, but results are variable and the preferred treatment for inoperable disease is chemotherapy, after which surgery may be possible or radiotherapy given to a smaller field causing fewer complications. Radiotherapy is particularly useful in the palliation of painful bony metastases and for preventing an impending paraplegia.

The majority of patients with neuroblastoma present with Stage IV disease and should be treated primarily with chemotherapy. Currently, the most effective treatment is to combine vincristine, cyclophosphamide and adriamycin. Although neuroblastoma is usually sensitive initially to chemotherapy, relapse occurs in the majority of patients within 6–12 months. Response to chemotherapy is reflected in a return of VMA excretion to normal and disappearance of neoplastic cells from the bone marrow.

The overall prognosis in neuroblastoma is poor (2-year survival rate is about 30 per cent). There is considerable variation, however, depending on the stage and age of patients. With Stage I disease the 2-year survival rate is over 80 per cent, but with Stage IV disease this falls to 5 per cent. The outlook for Stage IVS disease in infants under the age of one year is different and, despite the presence of distant metastases in the skin, liver and/or bone marrow (without radiological evidence of bone involvement), the 2-year survival is over 80 per cent. If patients survive for 2 years after primary treatment, without a recurrence of the disease, subsequent relapse is unusual and most of these patients are probably cured.

WILMS' TUMOUR (NEPHROBLASTOMA)

Wilms' tumour develops from cells of the embryonic mesonephric tissues and accounts for 20 per cent of childhood cancers. It has been believed that there is a particularly high incidence in children with a variety of congenital abnormalities (e.g. aniridia, hemihypertrophy, hypospadias, cryptorchidism, horse-shoe kidney, polycystic kidney and many other anomalies), suggesting a generalised developmental disorder, but recent reports have failed to confirm this.

Pathology

Wilms' tumour is characterised by rapid growth and the tumour may reach an exceptionally large size; it is often separated from the normal renal parenchyma by a pseudocapsule of thin connective tissue. The tumour invades locally to involve normal renal tissue and adjacent structures including the adrenal gland and diaphragm. There may also be direct extension along the ureters or the renal vein and inferior vena cava. Histologically, this tumour is usually cellular and poorly differentiated, but sometimes there is evidence of differentiation into glomeruli. The characteristic cell of the tumour is spindle-shaped and undifferentiated, resembling those in sarcomas. Wilms' tumour may show evidence of various other tissues of mesenchymal origin (for example fibrous tissue, adipose tissue, cartilage, bone or muscle).

Clinical features

90 per cent of cases of Wilms' tumour occur in children under the age of 8 and the peak incidence is between 2 and 4 years; on rare occasions it is clinically apparent at birth; in 5–10 per cent of cases both kidneys are affected. The usual presentation is of an enlarging abdomen, a smooth, hard, fixed mass being palpable, which may be of massive proportions occupying half the abdominal cavity. Excessive palpation should be avoided as there is evidence to suggest that this increases blood-borne dissemination. Pain is unusual, but may be caused either by haemorrhage into the abdominal cavity, or ureteric colic due to a blood clot or a piece of tumour in the ureter. Some patients have hypertension; and haematuria may occur. With the development of metastatic disease there is usually pallor, weight loss and anorexia. In 30 per cent of cases distant metastases are present at the time of diagnosis, the most common site to be affected being the lungs, but metastases may also develop in the liver, bones, pelvic organs, lymph nodes, mediastinum, pleural cavity and brain.

Wilms' tumour is staged according to the detectable extent of involvement:

Stage I	tumour limited to the kidney and completely resectable surgically;
Stage II	the tumour has extended beyond the kidney but is still completely resectable by surgery. e.g. there may be extension into the perirenal soft tissues, or para-aortic lymph-node involvement;
Stage III	tumour is confined to the abdomen, but residual tumour is left after surgery;
Stage IV	distant blood-borne metastases;
Stage V	bilateral renal involvement.

Investigations

The most important investigation is intravenous urography which characteristically demonstrates distortion of the calyceal pattern by the intrarenal mass. Occasionally, the tumour will not be demonstrable this way because the kidney has ceased to function, but it can then usually be demonstrated by retrograde pyelography. It is important that intravenous urography should show a functioning contra-lateral unaffected kidney, as Wilms' tumour has been described in solitary kidneys and such a finding would contra-indicate surgical excision of the tumour. Haematological and biochemical information may be of prognostic value; a high erythrocyte sedimentation rate is associated with a poor prognosis, elevation of the blood urea indicates impairment of renal function, and raised serum transaminases and alkaline phosphatase suggests the presence of hepatic metastases. Further evidence of metastatic disease may be gained by chest and skeletal radiography or isotopic bone scanning, while histological evidence of dissemination may be obtained by examination of bone marrow. The intravenous urogram is particularly valuable in differentiating Wilms' tumour from other abdominal but extra-renal tumours of childhood, particularly neuroblastoma.

Treatment

The modern management of Wilms' tumour has demonstrated how surgery, radiotherapy and chemotherapy can be combined in the initial management of a cancer to achieve a major improvement in cure rate. Surgical excision should be carried out first when feasible. It has been recommended that handling of tissues be gentle and that the renal pedicle is clamped before there is any manipulation of the tumour. Post-operative irradiation is given to the tumour bed. Pre-operative radiotherapy is reserved for those patients judged to be inoperable; after such treatment the tumour may be reduced to operable proportions and can then be removed. Because radiotherapy may affect vertebral bone growth, the field should be extended across the midline to include the whole of the vertebral bodies in order to prevent the development of scoliosis. It is important for the opposite kidney to be excluded completely from the radiation field. In addition to scoliosis and radiation nephritis, other possible adverse effects of radiotherapy are pulmonary fibrosis, if the lungs are irradiated for metastases, and the subsequent development of bone tumours. A recent trial has shown that post-operative radiotherapy can be omitted safely in patients aged less than 2 years with Stage I tumours.

The first cytotoxic drug to be effective in the treatment of metastatic Wilms' tumours was actinomycin D, and this remains the most effective drug. However, for Wilms' tumours resistant to actinomycin D, vincristine is of value and other drugs with activity include mustine, cyclophosphamide, nitrosoureas and adriamycin. It is now standard practice to treat children with this disease immediately with combination chemotherapy following operation. This has resulted in a marked decrease in the development of distant metastases and a striking improvement in survival. In Stage IV disease, chemotherapy is given as initial treatment until the disappearance, clinically, of pulmonary metastases, after which the primary tumour is excised and radiotherapy given to the renal bed and entire lungs.

When these tumours were treated by surgery alone the 5-year survival was about 15 per cent and the addition of post-operative irradiation increased this to 45 per cent. However, since the addition of adjuvant chemotherapy the 5-year survival has increased to over 80 per cent and it now seems probable that the majority of children with this tumour are curable.

HEPATOBLASTOMA

Hepatoblastoma is a rare embryonal tumour arising in the liver and associated with abnormally high levels of alpha foeto-protein in the blood in over 90 per cent of cases. Hepatoblastoma usually occurs before the age of three years when the presenting clinical features may include abdominal enlargement, pallor, weight loss, fever, anorexia, vomiting and diarrhoea; jaundice is uncommon. Vascular dissemination of this tumour occurs frequently; metastases being particularly common in the lungs.

The appropriate treatment for hepatoblastoma is surgical resection if feasible, but cure is rarely achieved. Hepatoblastoma is resistant to radiotherapy and the little information available on the use of chemotherapy is not encouraging.

PART 3

GENERAL MEDICAL ASPECTS

CHAPTER TWENTY

MALIGNANT EFFUSIONS

PLEURAL EFFUSION

Pathology

Primary mesotheliomas of the pleura cause effusions, but the majority of malignant pleural effusions are due to metastatic spread from other tissues, commonly from tumours of the breast, bronchus, ovary, gastro-intestinal tract or lymphomas. Metastatic nodules develop on the pleura with ulceration and exfoliation of malignant cells. Pleural fluid may also accumulate as a result of lymphatic obstruction in the chest wall or mediastinum, and, rarely, a chylous effusion may occur due to obstruction and rupture of the thoracic duct or one of its tributaries. Bronchial carcinoma may cause obstruction with pulmonary collapse and give rise to an effusion secondary to inflammatory changes. In the rare Meig's syndrome, fluid accumulates both in the peritoneal and pleural spaces in association with either a benign fibroma or malignant cystadenocarcinoma of the ovary.

Clinical features

Pleural effusion may be the most prominent symptomatic feature of malignant disease or an incidental part of more generalised disease. If large, dyspnoea and cough result and pain may be caused by infiltration of the chest wall. The clinical signs of pleural effusion are diminished movement on the affected side, absence of vocal fremitus, dullness to percussion and diminished breath sounds.

Investigations

The chest radiograph shows a homogenous opacity on the affected side(s), the extent depending upon the volume of fluid present. Metastases may also be visible in the lung, at the hilum, in the mediastinum and in the bones. Examination of the fluid shows that it is often macroscopically bloodstained in carcinoma of the lung, though this is rarely the case in effusions due to metastases from carcinoma of the breast. The presence of blood in the fluid is variable with other tumours. A chylous effusion resembles milk in appearance. Biochemical analysis of the fluid is seldom helpful in establishing the diagnosis, but cytological examination for malignant cells is valuable.

Treatment

The life expectancy of patients with metastatic pleural effusions may be prolonged, often many years, particularly in the case of breast cancer. Effective palliative treatment is therefore well worthwhile and a variety of methods exists. Aspiration or tube drainage alone leads in almost all instances to rapid re-accumulation of fluid unless effective antitumour treatment can be given concomitantly. Occasionally this may be radiotherapy, especially in the treatment of lymphomas, but this form of treatment is not feasible when metastatic involvement of the pleura is extensive. However, chemotherapy or hormone therapy in breast cancer can be successful in effecting control. Many tumours do not respond satisfactorily to the above methods and other treatment is then required to relieve discomfort and to avoid the necessity of repeated aspirations. The aim should be obliteration of the pleural space. All fluid should first be drained, full expansion of the lung achieved and a chemical pleuritis induced in order to obtain adhesion between the two pleural layers.

Adequate drainage is most readily achieved by the insertion of an intercostal catheter which is best placed in the axilla where the chest wall is relatively thin and a catheter causes least discomfort. Drainage should be gradual and is achieved by means of an under-water seal, the catheter remaining in place for several hours. When virtually all the fluid has been removed a chemical agent is instilled into the pleural space in order to produce an inflammatory reaction. Talc is probably the most effective, but this usually has to be given under a general anaesthetic, about 5 g being blown into the pleural space. However, this may be too exacting for a sick patient. Antimalarial drugs (mepacrine or quinacrine), tetracycline and silver nitrate have all been used but in our view mustine hydrochloride is at least as effective as anything else when 15–20 mg freshly dissolved in 50 ml of saline is instilled into the pleural space. The catheter is then clamped and the patient's position is altered during the next few minutes to allow the instilled fluid to flow over all of the pleural surfaces. The tube is then unclamped and drainage resumes until all fluid has been removed and the lung completely expanded; this may take up to 48 hours. This method has a high rate of success and recurrence of the effusion is unusual when the procedure has been undertaken with meticulous care. Occasionally, pleurectomy is performed, which produces obliteration of the pleural space and prevents accumulation of further fluid, but it is seldom needed and rarely justified in patients who are ill.

ASCITES

Primary mesotheliomas of the peritoneum cause ascites but, as with pleural mesotheliomas, these are rare. Peritoneal involvement by secondary deposits from primary tumours elsewhere is common, particularly adenocarcinomas from a variety of sites including the breast, bronchus, ovary and alimentary tract.

Ascites is caused by several mechanisms. Subserosal lymphatic obstruction is probably the most important factor, but there may be exudate from tumour nodules and increased permeability to albumen in the capillaries of the peritoneum. In some instances the same mechanism whereby ascites is produced in hepatic cirrhosis may operate, namely portal hypertension and hypoalbuminaemia. Pseudomyxoma peritonei is a rare condition in which pale mucilaginous material is found in the peritoneum ('mucinous ascites'). This is caused by ovarian tumours, usually mucinous cystadenomas or cystadenocarcinomas, though other ovarian, uterine and bowel tumours may be responsible. These tumours are either benign or of a low grade malignancy and do not metastasize but run a prolonged course. Chylous ascites, like a chylous pleural effusion, is caused by rupture of a lymphatic channel with accumulation of lymph in the peritoneum and, in a high proportion of cases, this is due to a malignant lymphoma. Other causes of ascites may have to be considered in a patient with malignant disease and these include Meig's syndrome (see above) and the development of bacterial peritonitis as a complication of the underlying illness.

Clinical features

The principal symptoms are abdominal distension, discomfort and sometimes pain with dyspnoea. Weight loss is variable because even if the patient is cachectic the accumulation of fluid may maintain body weight. Nausea and vomiting are common. The signs of ascites include distension centrally and in the flanks with eversion of the umbilicus. Shifting dullness and a fluid thrill can usually be detected by percussion. Examination of the fluid itself should be undertaken to establish the diagnosis. A relatively small volume (50–100 ml) can be aspirated through a small needle after infiltration of the skin, subcutaneous tissue and parietal peritoneum with local anaesthetic. It may appear bloodstained to the naked eye but is more usually clear. A protein content above 30 g per litre is an indication that it is an exudate and the specific gravity then usually exceeds 1.016. The level of glucose in the fluid is usually below 3.4 mmol/l and is often related to the number of free cells that are present. Cytological examination is a most helpful means of establishing with certainty the presence of metastatic disease, though it may sometimes be necessary to undertake peritoneoscopy.

Treatment

Prognosis of patients with malignant ascites is generally poor unless the tumour is responsive to systemic treatment as in the case of cancer of the breast. The treatment comprises generally palliative measures and aspiration of the fluid (paracentesis abdominis) is helpful but the fluid is likely to return rapidly unless concurrent systemic therapy is successful. It is occasionally effective to instil cytotoxic drugs into the peritoneum since these may kill tumour cells, thus reducing the tendency for fluid to collect, but this is not as successful as with pleural effusions. In many patients it is necessary to repeat paracentesis and it is often useful to give concurrent diuretic therapy including spironolactone.

In the rare instance of pseudomyxoma peritonei, surgical removal of the underlying tumour (ovary or appendix) and the peritoneal nodules, and evacuation of the mucinous material, followed by the instillation of an alkalating agent, may lead to a prolonged remission.

PERICARDIAL EFFUSION

Malignant pericardial effusions are less common than those of the pleural and peritoneal spaces. They are usually due to local spread from a carcinoma of the lung or breast but are also found as a late feature in a variety of other tumours. The tumour invades both parietal and visceral layers of the pericardium and may involve the myocardium. Interference with cardiac filling and constriction of the great veins occurs, leading ultimately to cardiac tamponade. Slow accumulation of fluid within the pericardial sac can produce a very large effusion.

Clinical features

A small pericardial effusion may cause no signs but, when it reaches moderate size, engorgement of the neck veins appears with an increase of venous pressure on inspiration (Kussmaul's sign). As the pressure within the pericardium increases the venous pressure rises and pulsation may disappear. Palpation of the arterial pulse and careful measurement of the blood pressure during inspiration and expiration shows increasing pulsus paradoxus which can become so pronounced that the pulse may disappear on inspiration. Other features include oedema in the legs and sacral area, a coarse rub over the praecordium, even when the effusion is large, and heart sounds reduced in intensity sometimes with an added (third) cardiac sound. A concurrent pleural effusion is often present.

Investigations

The electrocardiogram can be normal or may show low voltage complexes with deformity or inversion of the T wave throughout most leads and, occasionally, atrial fibrillation. A chest radiograph shows an increase in the cardiac outline with a sharply outlined border which can, however, be partly concealed by a pleural effusion. Echo-cardiography is the most valuable investigation and will usually indicate the presence of even a small pericardial effusion. Alternatively, a radioisotope technique may be used whereby the patient's red cells are labelled with technetium and re-injected into the circulation. The gamma camera records radio-activity over the blood-pools in the cavity of the heart and in the liver revealing, when a pericardial effusion is present, widening of the space between these two.

Treatment

The definitive management of a malignant pericardial effusion depends upon the nature of the underlying tumour. It may be necessary to remove fluid from the pericardium in order to relieve tamponade, but systemic treatment is needed to prevent a recurrence. This can be very successful in responsive tumours such as carcinoma of the breast and lymphomas but the prognosis with carcinoma of the lung is much worse.

Aspiration of a pericardial effusion is undertaken with the patient recumbent at an angle of approximately 45 degrees. The site of aspiration should be either between the xiphisternum and the left costal margin or through the anterior chest wall in the fifth left intercostal space 4–5 cm lateral to the sternal margin (in order to avoid the internal mammary vessels). If the pericardial effusion is large then it may be possible to aspirate safely from a wider area on the anterior chest wall. The skin and soft tissues including the parietal pleura should be infiltrated with lignocaine and a small stab incision made in the skin to allow easy entry of a large bore needle. Several types of needle or catheter are suitable but one of the easiest to use is the 'Longdwell' needle which projects through a teflon catheter with a Luer fitting and which is introduced on the end of a syringe. This is pushed gently backwards and slightly medially using the intercostal approach, but with the xiphisternal route the needle should be at an angle of 45 degrees to the skin and pointing towards the right sterno-clavicular joint. As the needle is advanced slowly, suction on the syringe will reveal when the pericardial sac has been entered. If a pleural effusion is present, this may be entered first by the intercostal approach and the needle can be advanced further. Malignant pericardial effusions are nearly always bloodstained and the inexperienced operator may be in doubt as to whether or not the heart has been entered. This can be decided by performing a haematocrit on a sample of the fluid aspirated. Some operators recommend attaching an electrocardiographic electrode to the needle when observation of a monitoring screen may indicate the characteristic complexes of an intra-cavity lead. In practice there is usually little difficulty when the effusion is large and the use of a soft catheter prevents the risk of damage to the heart. Fluid may be allowed to drain slowly into a sealed sterile plastic container or it may be aspirated either with a syringe or a low-vacuum pump. Removal of several hundred milli-litres may be achieved, with relief of the symptoms and signs.

CHAPTER TWENTY-ONE

METABOLIC DISORDERS

General metabolic disturbances occur in cancer patients, and these may be due to the effects of an advanced tumour, or more specifically they may be the result of involvement of particular organs by the tumour, or caused by its special biological properties.

Cachexia

Weight loss is an early feature in tumours of the upper gastro-intestinal tract when obstruction and ulceration make eating difficult. Anorexia is likely in most advanced tumours and although its mechanism is obscure it partly accounts for cachexia late in the disease. Other reasons for loss of weight are the rapid growth of some tumours at the expense of normal tissues, nausea and vomiting due to the disease, or sometimes its treatment, occasionally malabsorption, and often depression.

Hypercalcaemia

Hypercalcaemia occurs in about 10 per cent of patients with the commoner tumours but is found most frequently in carcinoma of the breast. There are two principal mechanisms. The usual cause is the presence of diffuse osteolytic skeletal metastases which by their growth displace large amounts of calcium into the blood. Less often, some tumours (mostly of the bronchus) produce a polypeptide resembling parathyroid hormone (see below) mobilising calcium from bones which are not necessarily the site of metastases. Regardless of the causative mechanism hypercalcaemia may be symptomless at first, but as the calcium level rises a variety of symptoms appear, and although this is usually a gradual process it may occasionally be rapid and dangerous.

Clinical features

The patient complains of lassitude, anorexia, nausea and constipation. Thirst and nocturia are frequently encountered and as the condition advances vomiting, dehydration, severe constipation and impairment of concentration may progress to drowsiness, frank psychosis and ultimately coma, renal failure and cardiac arrest. It is extremely important that these symptoms should be recognised and not ascribed to the underlying tumour since careful treatment can correct the plasma calcium level, reverse the symptoms and prevent death from this complication.

Although symptoms are plentiful, signs of hypercalcaemia are few.

There are likely to be features of dehydration but evidence of metastatic calcification should be sought in the eyes. Redness of the conjunctivae is common, particularly a horizontal leash of vessels extending from the limbus to the cornea. Deposits of calcium can often be seen as a thin, irregular white line where the cornea and sclera join laterally and medially (at 3 and 9 o'clock). It is necessary to examine the eye with a magnifying lens and in a strong light directed from the side.

Management

The aim of treatment is to replace fluid and to correct the level of plasma calcium. Since the patient is often nauseated, intravenous fluids may be required and about 4 litres daily should be given to achieve hydration and adequate urine flow. Oral phosphate given as buffered mixture of Na_2HPO_4 and $NaH_2PO_4H_2O$ to provide an intake of 3 g elemental phosphorus daily in three doses lowers the plasma calcium in two or three days. It may cause diarrhoea and be difficult to take if the patient is nauseated or vomiting. In these circumstances, and particularly in acute hypercalcaemia or when plasma calcium levels are very high, intravenous phosphate should be given. Phosphate lowers the calcium without increasing urinary excretion and probably produces extra-skeletal calcification. Corticosteroids are usually given although their effect upon the plasma calcium is unpredictable. Prednisolone 10 mg eight hourly is an adequate dose which can be reduced when the calcium levels return to normal. Other measures can be used but are not often necessary; these include diuretics (such as frusemide), mithramycin and calcitonin. In the longer term, specific treatment of the underlying tumour is the most appropriate method of controlling hypercalcaemia.

Hyperuricaemia

Hyperuricaemia is encountered most commonly in acute leukaemia but sometimes occurs in other malignant diseases. A rapid turnover of tumour cells leads to increased breakdown of nucleotides and elevation of the serum uric acid. Chemotherapy or radiotherapy may cause further increases. This may be accompanied by episodes of gout or, through precipitation of uric acid crystals in the renal tubules, obstructive nephropathy and anuria. Prevention of these events is best achieved by ensuring a high intake of fluid and by giving allopurinol 200–400 mg daily.

Hypoglycaemia

Hypoglycaemia occurs in association with certain tumours. Benign or malignant islet-cell tumours of the pancreas cause hypoglycaemia by producing increased amounts of insulin, but certain other tumours, notably hepatomas and large mesenchymal sarcomas, do so by means which are not understood. The demand for glucose by an enormous tumour is one probable explanation but depletion of certain enzymes (glucose-6-phosphatase and phosphorylase) in the liver can also occur.

Hepatic disorders

Liver metastases are very common when blood-borne spread has taken place. Numerous masses occur throughout the liver which are umbilicated on its surface. Spread to the peritoneum causes ascites which may be compounded by secondary hyperaldosteronism. Extensive metastases within the liver may cause portal hypertension and oesophageal varices, obstructive jaundice when the main bile ducts are occluded and, rarely, portal vein obstruction with subsequent thrombosis. In spite of the bulk of metastatic tumour, enough liver tissue remains to provide normal function until comparatively late. Jaundice is usually mild or absent unless occlusion of major bile ducts has occurred, and the stools tend to retain their normal colour. Complete obstruction of the bile ducts leads to pale stools and the presence of bile pigments in the urine.

Liver function tests may show only a slight increase in conjugated bilirubin and retention of bromsulphthalein. Later liver enzymes (alkaline phosphatase in particular, and transaminases) are increased and the serum globulin levels may be raised. In a wasted patient the serum albumin may be slightly reduced.

The importance of liver involvement lies in the prognosis, which, in the case of most tumours, usually becomes very bad. When liver function is impaired this necessitates modifications of drug therapy, particularly with cytotoxic agents such as cyclophosphamide, 5-fluorouracil and doxorubicin which are metabolised or excreted by the liver.

Renal disorders

Renal failure is seldom due to malignant disease except when pelvic and abdominal tumour masses cause ureteric obstruction or when calcium or uric acid are precipitated in the kidneys. Nephrocalcinosis follows prolonged hypercalcaemia but this is unusual in most cancers due to the short clinical course of the disease. Acute renal failure may occur in severe hypercalcaemia and as a result of uric acid crystals in the tubules. It occurs also in myelomatosis when the tubules may become obstructed by Bence–Jones protein. Most of these events can be anticipated and some prevented by methods described earlier, but impairment of renal function from any cause means that particular care should be taken in the use of all drugs, including cytotoxic agents.

Production of ectopic hormones

Ectopic hormones are polypeptides produced by a number of widely different tumours and which have biological activity similar to naturally occurring hormones. Production of large amounts of these polypeptides leads to well-recognised clinical syndromes.

Adrenocorticotrophic hormone (ACTH) is produced most often by oat-cell carcinomas of the bronchus but has been found in several other tumours including those of breast, gonads, pancreas and thyroid. The result of over stimulation of the adrenals is the appearance of Cushing's syndrome with diabetes, muscle weakness, hypokalaemia and hypertension. This form of the disease is found more frequently in men than women, the reverse of the type of Cushing's syndrome which is not due to ectopic ACTH. Plasma cortisol levels are very high and there is no diurnal variation. Occasionally, increased pigmentation is due to the simultaneous production of ectopic melanin-stimulating hormone. Treatment is difficult because the patient is usually seriously ill due to the underlying tumour. Bilateral adrenalectomy may occasionally be beneficial.

Parathyroid-like hormone may be produced by squamous-cell carcinoma of the bronchus in addition to tumours of the bowel, liver pancreas, kidney, uterus and, occasionally, by lymphomas. The result is hypercalcaemia (see above).

Antidiuretic hormone (vasopressin) is usually found in association with oat-cell bronchial carcinomas, and causes retention of water. This results in cellular overhydration which may lead to cerebral oedema and convulsions. The plasma sodium falls (often below 115 mmol/l) and plasma osmolality is lower than that of the urine. Treatment consists of restriction of water intake and giving fludrocortisone, while removal of the source of the ectopic hormone, if feasible, by resection or irradiation of the tumour, gives complete relief.

A large number of other ectopic hormone-producing tumours have been described but in practice these syndromes are rare.

CHAPTER TWENTY-TWO

INFECTIONS

Local or systemic infection causes serious illness and death in a large number of cancer patients. Local infection is likely to follow impaired drainage of, for example, the bronchial tubes, the genito-urinary tract or the bowel. Infections at these sites may indeed give rise to the presenting symptoms of a tumour and the response to treatment is likely to be poor unless the obstruction is relieved. For example, recurrent pneumonia is a well-known feature in carcinoma of the bronchus and is due to infection occurring distal to the obstructed lobar or segmental bronchus. Other consequences of tumours may be fistulae, leading to communications between the rectum and the bladder in tumours of these organs and of the cervix. Infection follows which is unlikely to improve until the fistula is closed. Skin infection may also occur where blood supply is impaired or where venous or lymphatic drainage is obstructed. An example of this is recurrent cellulitis occurring in the oedematous arm of some patients following radical mastectomy. Primary or metastatic tumours involving the skin or lymph nodes sometimes ulcerate, producing distressing necrotic areas which are difficult to heal.

Conditions predisposing to severe infection

Infections are the most important cause of death in patients with cancer. In patients with acute leukaemia approximately 70 per cent die as a result of pneumonia, septicaemia or some other serious infection. During the chemotherapy for induction of a remission in adults with leukaemia, approximately 60 per cent develop a serious infection and about a quarter of these die as a result. About half of patients with lymphomas, myeloma and solid tumours eventually develop fatal infections. Most of these are bacterial, a small number being caused by fungi. Although viral infections are relatively common they are usually not fatal.

Neutropenia is responsible for frequent infections in cancer patients. It is commonly encountered in haematological malignancies and inter-mittently in patients treated with cytotoxic chemotherapy. Not only may the number of granulocytes be reduced to a level at which infection is likely to occur and to be severe, but the function of these cells is also impaired in leukaemias and in Hodgkin's disease. Disturbances of immune mechanisms increase susceptibility to infection in two ways. In chronic lymphocytic leukaemia, lymphocytic lymphoma and myelomatosis, there is impaired production of antibodies. In Hodgkin's disease, however, there is impairment of cellular immunity, making patients liable to certain bacterial and fungal infections. Although not as important as granulocytopenia, lymphopenia also occurs in certain malignancies and is associated with an increased risk of infection.

During chemotherapy a number of consequences make patients more susceptible to bacterial invasion, including ulceration of the mucous membranes (allowing organisms to penetrate the wall of the gut), leukopenia and inhibition of immunological responses. Antibiotic therapy may influence the ultimate infection by altering the normal flora of the intestine and skin and producing resistant strains which are later more difficult to treat. Major surgery is followed by non-specific interference with resistance to infection, while splenectomy can be followed by fulminating bacterial infection. Radiotherapy may similarly impair immune responses.

Although these factors indicate why patients with cancer are more liable to infection, there are other considerations which determine both the site and type of infection. Pneumonia and septicaemia are encountered more often in patients with leukaemias than any other form of malignancy. Nevertheless, primary or secondary tumours of the lung, cancers of the head and neck, especially where major surgery has been undertaken with formation of a tracheostomy, all predispose to the development of pneumonia. Septicaemia is particularly likely to occur with tumours of the genito-urinary tract and of the bowel. The single most important factor, however, which determines whether otherwise innocuous organisms or a trivial infection produces life-threatening septicaemia is neutropenia, especially when the total white-cell count falls well below $10^9/l$.

The presence of a catheter in the bladder for any length of time virtually ensures infection of the urinary tract and reconstructive surgery with the formation of an ileal conduit makes the patient vulnerable to infection. A breach in the surface of the skin is an important source of organisms through superficial ulcers or prolonged intravenous infusions.

It is important to remember that in neutropenic patients any infection may spread widely and rapidly if treatment is not instituted without delay. Moreover the classical symptoms and signs usually associated with infection may be absent or masked. In patients with cancer more than any others and particularly in the presence of neutropenia, gram-negative septicaemia is common, and fatal if not treated promptly.

Bacterial infections

About 70 per cent of fatal infections in patients with acute leukaemia are due to bacteria and an even greater proportion in patients with solid tumours. The organisms most often responsible are virulent gram-negative bacilli but even bacteria not normally pathogenic, such as *Staphylococcus epidermidis*, can be dangerous in the neutropenic patient. The three organisms most frequently encountered are *Pseudomonas aeruginosa, Escherichia coli* and *Klebsiella pneumoniae*. *P. aeruginosa* is found universally in hospitals, particularly in moist areas near taps, pipes and in tubing. It is likely to cause bronchopneumonia, skin infections and may infect the eye, meninges and gut. *K. pneumoniae* causes serious respiratory tract infection or septicaemia. *E. coli* infection is common and this organism can gain entry to the circulation from the intestine. A great variety of other organisms may cause infections but these are less common. They include Clostridia, Salmonellae and occasionally *M. tuberculosis*.

Treatment

It is preferable to use bactericidal antibiotics, the penicillins being particularly effective against susceptible organisms. Staphylococcal infections require benzylpenicillin, flucloxacillin or fusidic acid according to sensitivity of the organism. Gram-negative infections should be treated in accordance with laboratory reports of sensitivity and intravenous therapy is essential. Gentamycin is initially the antibiotic of choice, usually combined with ampicillin; cotrimoxazole or a cephalosporin are also useful.

In the case of infections due to *P. aeruginosa* carbenicillin in large doses (5 g four hourly) should be given together with gentamycin. Because of the serious, rapidly fatal course of gram-negative infections in cancer patients, the onset of any fever requires rapid action. Blood cultures should be obtained immediately and then empirical treatment begun before the results are known.

Fungal infections

Infections caused by a variety of fungi are being recognised more commonly in cancer patients and these 'opportunistic' infections have the same predisposing conditions as the bacterial infections mentioned above. Fungi which do not usually cause infection in healthy patients can be responsible for serious and fatal illness when host defences are impaired. These include *Candida* and *Aspergillus* species, particularly in acute leukaemias. Some other fungal infections tend to occur naturally in certain parts of the world among the healthy general population and these are not seen any more often in patients with cancer but may give rise to disseminated infection when a previously healed lesion becomes reactivated. This is liable to happen in patients with lymphomas and the fungi responsible are *Cryptococcus neoformans, Nocardia asteroides* and, in North America, *Histoplasma capsulatum* and *Coccidioides immitus*.

Candida is the most common fungal infection in patients with cancer and may involve the skin, the mouth and pharynx or, later, the intestinal tract, lungs and ultimately become a systemic infection. For local infection of the skin Nystatin applied topically in the form of a powder or cream is effective. In the mouth a Nystatin suspension given as a mouth wash and then swallowed, or Nystatin lozenges sucked at 4 hourly intervals, is usually followed by healing within a few days. The flavour of Nystatin, however, is so disagreeable that amphotericin B lozenges which are usually equally effective and very much more palatable are preferred. For severe infection of the oesophagus and intestine, in addition to the above measures, amphotericin tablets should be swallowed at 4 hourly intervals and may be supplemented by an intravenous infusion of amphotericin B for up to seven days. Pulmonary candidiasis usually takes the form of diffuse pneumonia and treatment is seldom effective. Disseminated candidiasis may be treated by an intravenous infusion of amphotericin B or by 5-fluorocytosine which is less nephrotoxic.

Aspergillus infections involving the lung and other parts of the respiratory tract, including the sinuses, are being seen more often. They are difficult to recognise but tend to occur in patients with leukaemias and lymphomas, particularly during treatment with chemotherapy, corticosteroids and antibiotics. Proof of the diagnosis is difficult to obtain during life, and although it is worth trying the effect of amphotericin or 5-fluorocytosine, treatment is usually ineffective.

Viral infections

Viruses can cause severe infections in patients with cancer but they are less often life-threatening than those caused by bacteria. DNA virus infections are the commonest and of these cytomegalic inclusion disease is one of the more important. It is caused by the cytomegalovirus (C.M.V.), a herpes simplex-like virus which causes patchy bilateral pneumonia. Another common cause of infection is the varicella virus which produces herpes zoster, sometimes occurring in the dermatome supplied by a nerve root close to a tumour or the site of previous radiotherapy. It is particularly common in Hodgkin's disease and other lymphomas and may either give rise to localised shingles or a disseminated infection resembling chicken pox. Very early treatment with local applications of idoxuridine or intravenous adenine arabinoside may abort an attack of herpes zoster.

Herpes simplex infections involve the lips, nose, mouth or cause dendritic ulcers in the cornea. These lesions may become secondarily infected with bacteria and cause considerable mutilation. Generalised vaccinia, which is often fatal, is likely to occur in immunosuppressed patients, particularly those with leukaemias or lymphomas who are vaccinated against smallpox. Fatalities are sometimes prevented by giving vaccinia–immune globulin.

Other viruses may be responsible for illness in patients with compromised immunity, among these being the hepatitis A and B and measles viruses.

Protozoal infections

Protozoal infections are uncommon but *Pneumocystis carinii* pneumonia is seen in patients with lymphomas and leukaemias or in those who have received chemotherapy and antibiotics. Characteristically, this infection produces bilateral pulmonary shadowing on the chest radiograph due to a patchy pneumonia. The patient complains of cough and increasing dyspnoea which develops over the course of several days. The disease is rapidly fatal unless treated with either pentamidine or large doses of cotrimoxazole.

Prophylactic measures

Serious infections may be reduced by taking preventative measures. By nursing severely leukopenic patients in isolation, using reversed barrier precautions, and incorporating certain physical devices to protect them from external organisms, the frequency of infection can be reduced. Such measures are elaborate, expensive and not generally available. They include the use of rooms with laminar air flow so that dust and micro-organisms are trapped in a filter and excluded from the circulating air. Alternatively, the patient can be nursed enclosed in a form of plastic tent or curtain which has ports in the side fitted with gloves allowing procedures to be undertaken by the medical and nursing staff. Since endogenous micro-organisms are the source of many infections these can be reduced by giving non-absorbed broad-spectrum antibiotics by mouth and by bathing the patients using bactericidal soap. Topical antibiotics will remove organisms from the perineum and other areas of skin and if food is sterilised, new micro-organisms are prevented from entering the gut.

In practice, most of the above prophylactic measures are only possible in a few specialised centres. Fortunately, the short periods of granulocytopenia that are frequently encountered during chemotherapy, and which are followed by prompt recovery of the blood count, are usually safe. Many patients in these circumstances remain at home (where they are probably exposed to fewer noxious organisms than in hospital) but even those in general wards do not develop serious infections provided the marrow recovers within 2–3 days. More prolonged neutropenia does require management in protected surroundings.

CHAPTER TWENTY-THREE

SYMPTOMATIC AND SUPPORTIVE CARE

The survey of individual tumours in Part 2 indicates that malignancy may be associated with a wide variety of medical disturbances. These must receive attention if the best results of specific antitumour therapy are to be obtained.

Pain is probably the most common symptom in advanced cancer, but if the tumour responds to its specific therapy, it may be a temporary feature. With cancers refractory to treatment, pain may become permanent and progressively more severe. Its intensity is affected greatly by the patient's mood and morale. A wide variety of analgesic preparations are available, but attention must also be paid to anxiety and depression which have a marked effect on pain threshold. Mild pain can generally be controlled satisfactorily by oral analgesics (e.g. paracetamol alone or combined with dextropropoxyphene; aspirin alone or in various compound tablets). Should these preparations be insufficient to control pain then more powerful analgesics such as codeine, dihydrocodeine, dextromoramide and methadone may be needed and more severe pain requires opium derivatives, the best being diamorphine. In the dying patient the problem of addiction is irrelevant.

Persistent pain is controlled more effectively by analgesic drugs administered at regular times; it is generally undesirable to prescribe analgesics on an 'as required' basis. A patient's requirement for analgesia should be judged carefully and the appropriate dose given with the correct frequency to control pain without interruption. In patients with long and painful terminal illnesses, it is often useful to give analgesics in combination with other drugs in the form of a palatable syrup which permits the strength of the constituents to be varied. Several such mixtures are available containing combinations of morphine, diamorphine, cocaine and chloroform water or alcohol. Because opiate drugs may induce nausea, it is sometimes of value to add a phenothiazine (prochlorperazine or chlorpromazine) to these mixtures. Bone pain is sometimes treated effectively with anti-inflammatory drugs (aspirin, indomethacin, naproxen) and it is possible that these drugs act by inhibiting prostaglandins which may be responsible for mediating lysis of bone in the presence of metastases. Localised bone pain can usually be treated adequately by radiotherapy.

Skeletal metastases may be so extensive as to compromise bone-marrow function, in a way that is similar to primary bone-marrow tumours (leukaemias, myelomatosis). Characteristically, there is a leukoerythroblastic blood picture in which immature blood cells are present in the peripheral blood. Severe anaemia may develop, leukopenia may lead to infection, and thrombocytopenia can result in purpura or serious bleeding. Anaemia is corrected by blood transfusion, neutropenia and associated infections should be treated with appropriate antibiotics (Chapter 22). In the acute leukaemias, in which severe marrow suppression may result both from the disease and the treatment, it is sometimes of value to give leukocyte transfusions. Thrombocytopenia associated with osseous metastases can be reversed by administering vincristine, which is often effective alone, but the addition of corticosteroids may enhance this effect. After platelet stimulation in this way, definitive antitumour treatment previously not possible may then be practicable (e.g. hypophysectomy; myelosuppressive chemotherapy). Bleeding secondary to severe thrombocytopenia should be treated with transfusions of fresh platelets.

Other complications of skeletal metastases include hypercalcaemia (Chapter 21) and a liability to pathological fractures. Such fractures may need orthopaedic surgical procedures. It is preferable, however, for fractures of weight-bearing bones to be anticipated and a pin or plate inserted prophylactically. Radiotherapy to osseous metastases is often effective in preventing fractures, and irradiation of spinal metastases may stop vertebral collapse and a paraplegia from occurring. Further discussion of neurological complications of malignant disease is given elsewhere (Chapter 17). Patients with skeletal complications may have to undergo long periods of immobilisation, particularly after some surgical procedures, but may, for example with breast cancer, have subsequently a good chance of response to specific antitumour therapy. Such patients need much encouragement and help to regain function and in these circumstances physiotherapists play an essential role.

Dyspnoea, complicating malignant disease, may be caused by pleural or pericardial effusions (Chapter 20) or pulmonary infiltration by the tumour. In the latter case, alleviation usually depends on the response of the tumour to specific therapy, but occasionally bronchodilators, such as salbutamol or corticosteroids, are of value. When pulmonary infections contribute to dyspnoea, appropriate antibiotics may be used, but if the underlying malignant disease is untreatable this may only serve to prolong a terminal illness. Various linctuses are available to treat cough; codeine or pholcodeine are usually adequate initially, but for more severe or intractable coughing methadone or diamorphine linctus is necessary.

Nausea and vomiting in cancer patients may be due to the underlying disease, to some of its complications (e.g. hypercalcaemia) or to therapy (e.g. cytotoxic drugs, radiotherapy). Phenothiazine derivatives, particularly prochlorperazine or chlorpromazine, and metoclopromide are valuable anti-emetic drugs. Anorexia sometimes accompanies malignant disease, and in this case small doses of corticosteroids or moderate quantities of preprandial alcohol may be useful to stimulate the appetite.

Dry mouth is a frequent complication of radiotherapy in the head and neck region, and this may be caused by certain drugs or result simply from dehydration. Dehydration should, if possible, be prevented but in the normally hydrated patient a dry mouth can be effectively relieved by mouth washes of 'artificial saliva' (a methylcellulose-based preparation) before meals. Stomatitis and oral ulceration may be caused by certain cytotoxic drugs. This should usually be avoided by careful calculation of drug dosages based on detailed familiarity with their actions and the patient's metabolic function relevant to drug metabolism. (e.g. renal function with methotrexate, liver function with adriamycin). Salicylate mouth washes may relieve symptoms from oral ulceration, and super-infection with Candida should be treated by amphotericin or Nystatin mouth washes and lozenges. If these complications interfere with the patient's ability to take nutrition it may be necessary to institute, temporarily, nasogastric or intravenous feeding. However, such measures are inappropriate if they would merely prolong an unpleasant terminal illness.

Pruritus may be associated with obstructive jaundice, while occasion-ally it is a general manifestation of malignancy, particularly Hodgkin's disease, in which case its mechanism is obscure. Pruritus may be difficult to relieve but, when associated with biliary stasis, cholestyramine may help; other drugs which may be tried include antihistamines, such as promethazine or chlorpheniramine, phenobarbitone or corticosteroids.

Fungating growths can be extremely distressing and need careful nursing care. The offensiveness of these lesions may be mitigated by Nilodor incorporated in dressings or, as anerobes are often responsible, systemic metronidazole.

Of all maladies, cancer is one of the most emotive in engendering fear in patients. However, even cancers which are not curable may be associated with many years of life. During such prolonged, chronic diseases patients are liable to have periods of anxiety or depression. Anxiety states are suitably treated by mild tranquillizers, such as diazepam, but these should not be given in the presence of depression as this may be aggravated by these drugs. Depression should be treated specifically with tricyclic antidepressants (e.g. amitriptyline, imipramine, protriptyline). It is important for medical and nursing staff to recognise psychiatric dis-turbances and give patients ample opportunity for their problems to be discussed and reassurance to be given. A truthful explanation about the illness should always be given to patients, as not to do so may lead to difficulties in the future. A patient may lose confidence if he or she believes that information is being withheld or incorrect explanations have been given. By the same token, it is not required for a medical attendant to volunteer all details in a thoroughly candid fashion if this has not been requested; such unsolicited information may itself cause the patient considerable distress unnecessarily. It is, therefore, important for a correct balance to be achieved for each individual patient. Close relatives should be aware of a patient's prognosis and be encouraged to give appropriate support and have a forthright approach to their sick relatives so that an atmosphere of honesty can exist and embarrassment avoided. As cancer treatment improves and the word 'cancer' becomes less associated with fear and despondency, society will find it easier to face these problems.

FURTHER READING

1. J. F. Holland and E. Frei (eds), *Cancer Medicine*, Lea and Febiger, Philadelphia, 1974.
   A comprehensive textbook covering all aspects of oncology.
2. J. Horton and G. J. Hill, (eds), *Clinical Oncology*, W. B. Saunders, Philadelphia, London, Toronto, 1977.
   Another useful comprehensive textbook, less exhaustive than the above.
3. K. D. Bagshawe (ed.), *Medical Oncology—Medical Aspects of Malignant Disease*, Blackwell Scientific Publications, Oxford, 1975.
   Detailed coverage of selected oncological subjects.
4. A. Clarysse, Y. Kenis and G. Mathé, *Cancer Chemotherapy—Its Role in the Treatment Stategy of Haematologic Malignancies and Solid Tumours*, Springer-Verlag Berlin, Heidelberg, New York, 1976.
   A detailed, up to date account of all aspects of the systemic treatment of cancer.
5. S. Lowery, *Fundamentals of Radiation Therapy*, Hodder and Stoughton Educational, Sevenoaks, 1974.
   A short textbook on the principles of radiotherapy.
6. Cicely Saunders (ed.), *Management of Terminal Disease*, Edward Arnold, London, 1978.
   An account of patient care during the terminal stages of illness.

INDEX